Arthroscopy of the Foot and Ankle

Editor

LAURENCE RUBIN

CLINICS IN PODIATRIC MEDICINE AND SURGERY

www.podiatric.theclinics.com

Consulting Editor
THOMAS J. CHANG

July 2023 • Volume 40 • Number 3

ELSEVIER

1600 John F. Kennedy Boulevard • Suite 1800 • Philadelphia, Pennsylvania, 19103-2899

http://www.theclinics.com

CLINICS IN PODIATRIC MEDICINE AND SURGERY Volume 40, Number 3
July 2023 ISSN 0891-8422, ISBN-13: 978-0-323-96151-6

Editor: Megan Ashdown
Developmental Editor: Arlene Campos

Clinics in Podiatric Medicine and Surgery (ISSN 0891-8422) is published quarterly by Elsevier Inc., 360 Park Avenue South, New York, NY 10010-1710. Months of issue are January, April, July, and October. Business and Editorial Offices: 1600 John F. Kennedy Blvd., Ste. 1800, Philadelphia, PA 19103-2899. Customer Service Office: 3251 Riverport Lane, Maryland Heights, MO 63043. Periodicals postage paid at New York, NY and additional mailing offices. Subscription prices are $329.00 per year for US individuals, $625.00 per year for US institutions, $100.00 per year for US students and residents, $405.00 per year for Canadian individuals, $754.00 for Canadian institutions, $490.00 for international individuals, $754.00 per year for international institutions, $100.00 per year for Canadian students/residents, and $220.00 per year for foreign students/residents. To receive student/resident rate, orders must be accompanied by name of affiliated institution, date of term, and the *signature* of program/residency coordinator on institution letterhead. Orders will be billed at individual rate until proof of status is received. Foreign air speed delivery is included in all *Clinics* subscription prices. All prices are subject to change without notice. POSTMASTER: Send address changes to *Clinics in Podiatric Medicine and Surgery*, Elsevier Health Sciences Division, Subscription Customer Service, 3251 Riverport Lane, Maryland Heights, MO 63043. **Customer Service: 1-800-654-2452 (US). From outside of the US, call 314-447-8871. Fax: 314-447-8029. E-mail: JournalsCustomerService-usa@elsevier.com (for print support); JournalsOnlineSupport-usa@elsevier.com (for online support).**

Reprints. For copies of 100 or more of articles in this publication, please contact the Commercial Reprints Department, Elsevier Inc., 360 Park Avenue South, New York, NY 10010-1710. Tel.: 212-633-3874; Fax: 212-633-3820; E-mail: reprints@elsevier.com.

Clinics in Podiatric Medicine and Surgery is covered in *MEDLINE/PubMed (Index Medicus)* and *EMBASE/Excerpta Medica*.

Contributors

CONSULTING EDITOR

THOMAS J. CHANG, DPM
Clinical Professor and Past Chairman, Department of Podiatric Surgery, CCPM Faculty, The Podiatry Institute, Sonoma County Orthopedic/Podiatric Specialists, Santa Rosa, California

EDITOR

LAURENCE RUBIN, DPM, FACFAS
Private Practice, Richmond, Virginia; Past President, American College of Foot and Ankle Surgeons, Director, Virginia Fellowship in Reconstruction, Revision, and Limb Preservation Surgery of the Foot and Ankle, Foot and Ankle Specialists of Virginia, Mechanicsville, Virginia

AUTHORS

TROY J. BOFFELI, DPM, FACFAS
Director, Foot and Ankle Surgical Residency Program, Regions Hospital/HealthPartners Institute, TRIA Woodbury Orthopedic Center, Chair, Foot and Ankle Surgery, HealthPartners Medical Group, Saint Paul, Minnesota

PHILLIP M. CALAJ, DPM
Resident Physician, Department of Podiatric Surgery, Advent Health East Orlando Podiatric Surgery Residency, Orlando, Florida

MEAGAN COLEMAN, DPM, AACFAS
Past Fellow, Orthopaedic Institute Brielle Orthopedics, Manasquan, New Jersey

JAMES COTTOM, DPM, FACFAS
Director, Florida Orthopedic Foot and Ankle Center Fellowship, Sarasota, Florida

BRIAN DERNER, DPM, AACFAS
Fellow, The CORE Institute Reconstructive Foot and Ankle Fellowship, The CORE Institute, Phoenix, Arizona

RICHARD DERNER, DPM, FACFAS
Residency Director, INOVA Fairfax Medical Center, Fairfax, Virginia

LAWRENCE DIDOMENICO, DPM, FACFAS
Director, Reconstructive Rearfoot and Ankle Fellowship, NOMS Ankle and Foot Care Center, Youngstown, Ohio; Director, East Liverpool City Hospital Residency Program, East Liverpool, Ohio

MICHAEL D. DUJELA, DPM, FACFAS
Fellowship Trained Foot and Ankle Surgeon, Director, Advanced Reconstructive Foot and Ankle Surgery Fellowship, Washington Orthopaedic Center, Centralia, Washington

FRANK FELIX, DPM
Second Year Podiatric Medicine and Surgery Resident, Baylor Scott and White Memorial Hospital, Texas A&M Health Science Center, Temple, Texas

THOMAS D. FERRISE, DPM
Resident Physician, Department of Podiatric Surgery, Advent Health East Orlando Podiatric Surgery Residency, Orlando, Florida

SAMANTHA M. FIGAS, DPM, AACFAS
Podiatric Surgery Specialist, Department of Orthopaedic Surgery, Cleveland Clinic, Akron General, Akron, Ohio

SEAN T. GRAMBART, DPM, FACFAS
Assistant Dean of Clinical Affairs, Des Moines University College of Podiatric Medicine and Surgery, Attending, IMMC Foot and Ankle Surgery Residency Program, Des Moines, Iowa

JORDAN P. GROSSMAN, DPM, FACFAS
Chief, Section of Podiatry, Cleveland Clinic, Akron General, Akron, Ohio

SHANE HOLLAWELL, DPM, FACFAS
Fellowship Director, Orthopaedic Institute Brielle Orthopedics, Manasquan, New Jersey

NATHANIEL HOLTE, DPM
Resident, IMMC Foot and Ankle Surgery Residency Program, Des Moines, Iowa

BRIAN E. HOUNG, DPM, MS, AACFAS
Fellow, Advanced Reconstructive Foot and Ankle Surgery, Washington Orthopedic Center, Centralia, Washington

MICHAEL S. LEE, DPM, FACFAS
Foot and Ankle Surgeon, Capital Orthopaedics & Sports Medicine PC, Clive, Iowa

JOHN A. MARTUCCI, DPM, AACFAS
Fellow, Reconstructive Rearfoot and Ankle Fellowship, NOMS Ankle and Foot Care Center, Youngstown, Ohio

SAMANTHA A. MINER, DPM, AACFAS
Fellow, Reconstructive Foot and Ankle Fellowship, Coordinated Health/Lehigh Valley Health Network, Bethlehem, Pennsylvania

ALAN NG, DPM, FACFAS
Physician, Foot and Ankle Surgery, Advanced Orthopedics & Sports Medicine Specialists, Orthopedic Centers of Colorado, Denver, Colorado

GARRETT B. NGUYEN, DPM
Chief Resident Physician, Department of Podiatric Surgery, Advent Health East Orlando Podiatric Surgery Residency, Orlando, Florida

KEVIN NGUYEN, DPM, AACFAS
Podiatric Surgeon Fellow, Advanced Orthopedics & Sports Medicine Specialists, Orthopedic Centers of Colorado, Denver, Colorado

ALIVIA PASSET, DPM
Resident, IMMC Foot and Ankle Surgery Residency Program, Des Moines, Iowa

MADISON RAVINE, DPM
Resident Physician, Cambridge Health Alliance Podiatric Medicine and Surgery
Residency Program, Cambridge, Massachusetts

CHRISTOPHER L. REEVES, DPM, FACFAS
Faculty, Advent Health East Orlando Podiatric Surgery Residency, Director of Research,
Advent Health East Orlando Podiatric Surgery Residency, Rothman Orthopaedic Institute,
Orlando, Florida

LAURENCE RUBIN, DPM, FACFAS
Private Practice, Richmond, Virginia; Past President, American College of Foot and Ankle
Surgeons, Director, Virginia Fellowship in Reconstruction, Revision, and Limb
Preservation Surgery of the Foot and Ankle, Foot and Ankle Specialists of Virginia,
Mechanicsville, Virginia

RYAN T. SCOTT, DPM, FACFAS
Director, The CORE Institute Reconstructive Foot and Ankle Fellowship, The CORE
Institute, Phoenix, Arizona

AMBER M. SHANE, DPM, FACFAS
Chair, Department of Podiatric Surgery Advent Health System, Faculty, Advent Health
East Orlando Podiatric Surgery Residency, Medical Director, Upperline Health, Orlando,
Florida

NAOHIRO SHIBUYA, DPM, MS
Clinical Professor, University of Texas Rio Grande Valley, School of Podiatric Medicine,
Edinburg, Texas

ALDEN SIMMONS, DPM
Third Year Podiatric Medicine and Surgery Resident, Baylor Scott and White Memorial
Hospital, Texas A&M Health Science Center, Temple, Texas

JONATHON SROUR, DPM, AACFAS
Double Fellowship-Trained Foot and Ankle Surgeon, Tier 1 Orthopedic and Neurosurgical
Institute, Cookeville, Tennessee

TYLER TEWILLIAGER, DPM, AACFAS
Fellowship Trained Podiatric Foot and Ankle Surgeon, Advanced Orthopedics & Sports
Medicine Specialists, Orthopedic Centers of Colorado, Denver, Colorado

MICHAEL H. THEODOULOU, DPM, FACFAS
Division Chief, Podiatric Surgery, Cambridge Health Alliance, Assistant Professor of
Surgery, Harvard Medical School, Cambridge, Massachusetts

JONATHAN C. THOMPSON, DPM, MHA, FACFAS
Foot and Ankle Surgeon, Division of Orthopedics, Mayo Clinic Health System, Eau Claire,
Wisconsin

BEN M. TONSAGER, DPM
Resident, Foot and Ankle Surgical Residency Program, Regions Hospital, HealthPartners
Institute, Saint Paul, Minnesota

ARJUN VIJAYAKUMAR, DPM
Resident Physician, Kaiser Permanente South Bay Consortium, Santa Clara, California

GLENN M. WEINRAUB, DPM, FACFAS
Attending Physician, Department of Orthopaedic Surgery, Kaiser Permanente, San Leandro, California

JOSEPH WOLF, DPM, AACFAS
Foot and Ankle Surgeon, Ohio Foot and Ankle Specialists, Sylvania, Ohio

JOSHUA WOLFE, DPM, MHA, AACFAS
Fellow, The CORE Institute Reconstructive Foot and Ankle Fellowship, The CORE Institute, Phoenix, Arizona

SARA YANCOVITZ, DPM, AACFAS
Fellow, Orthopaedic Institute Brielle Orthopedics, Manasquan, New Jersey

Contents

A wide spectrum of pathologies can lead to soft tissue abnormalities within the ankle joint. Many of these disorders can develop into irreversible joint degeneration if left untreated. Arthroscopy is frequently used to treat these soft tissue conditions such as instability, synovitis, impingement, arthrofibrosis, and other inflammatory disorders in the rearfoot and ankle. In general, the etiology of these ankle soft tissue disorders can be classified as traumatic, inflammatory, and congenital/neoplastic. Overall, the goal of diagnosing and treating soft tissue pathologies of the ankle is to restore anatomic and physiologic motion, reduce pain, optimize functional return to activity, and decrease the chance of recurrence while minimizing complications.

Arthroscopic reduction of tibiotalar osteophytes results in good to excellent results in the vast majority of patients. Pain is primarily due to synovial hypertrophy and anterior tibiotalar entrapment associated with the osteophytes. Osteophytes may be due to repetitive trauma such as sports, or associated with subtle or overt ankle instability. A minimally invasive approach results in rapid recovery and less risk than open interventions. In cases where anterior osteophytes have coexisting ankle instability and in many cases ancillary procedures such as ankle stabilization are performed.

This article is devoted to managing posterior ankle impingement syndrome and its management using endoscopic to arthroscopic surgical instrumentation. The authors explore the critical anatomy, pathogenesis, and clinical examination. Operative techniques, including the approach, and instrumentation used, are outlined. The postoperative protocol is discussed. Finally, a literature review is provided, which also defines known complications.

with an open procedure. In particular, posterior arthroscopic subtalar joint arthrodesis (PASTA) allows a reproducible and viable alternative to standard lateral-portal subtalar joint (STJ) arthrodesis without violating sinus or canalis tarsi neurovascular structures. Additionally, those patients who have undergone previous total ankle arthroplasty, arthrodesis, or talonavicular joint arthrodesis may be better served with PASTA over open arthrodesis if STJ fusion becomes necessary. This article describes the unique PASTA surgical procedure and its helpful tips and pearls.

Arthroscopic cartilage repair has made several strides in recent years; however, no gold standard for cartilage restoration has been found. Simple treatment with bone marrow stimulation such as microfracture have shown good short-term results; however, concerns for long-term stability of cartilage repair as well as the subchondral bone health remain in question. Treatment of these lesions often comes down to surgeon preference, the aim of this study is to discuss some of the current options available on the market to further assist surgeons in their decision-making process.

The indications and procedures for arthroscopy of the ankle and subtalar joints continues to increase. Lateral ankle instability is a common pathology that may require surgery to repair injured structures of patients nonresponsive to conservative management. Common surgical methods generally include ankle arthroscopy with subsequent open approach to repair/reconstruct the ankle ligament(s). This article discusses two different approaches to repairing lateral ankle instability through an arthroscopic approach. The arthroscopic modified Brostrom procedure creates a strong repair with minimal soft tissue dissection, and is a reliable, minimally invasive approach to lateral ankle stabilization. The arthroscopic double ligament stabilization procedure creates a robust reconstruction of the anterior talofibular and calcaneal fibular ligaments with minimal soft tissue dissection.

Alongside advances and trends in foot and ankle surgery, arthroscopy provides a minimally invasive option in exploring and addressing pain after total ankle replacement (TAR). It is not uncommon for patients to develop pain months or even years after TAR implantation for both fixed and mobile-bearing designs. Arthroscopic debridement of gutter pain can provide successful outcomes in the hands of the experienced arthroscopist. Surgeon preference and experience will dictate the threshold for intervention, approach, and tool selection. This article provides a brief look into the background, indications, technique, limitations, and outcomes for arthroscopy after TAR.

CLINICS IN PODIATRIC MEDICINE AND SURGERY

SERIES OF RELATED INTEREST

Orthopedic Clinics
https://www.orthopedic.theclinics.com/
Clinics in Sports Medicine
https://www.sportsmed.theclinics.com/
Foot and Ankle Clinics
https://www.foot.theclinics.com/
Physical Medicine and Rehabilitation Clinics
https://www.pmr.theclinics.com/

THE CLINICS ARE AVAILABLE ONLINE!
Access your subscription at:
www.theclinics.com

Foreword

Arthroscopy Foreword

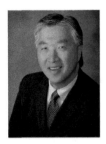

Thomas J. Chang, DPM
Consulting Editor

During my residency training in 1990, Arthroscopy was done primarily in the ankle joint, treating osteochondral injuries and other inflammatory conditions. I went to my first course with ACFAS in Chicago and was excited to explore this rapidly growing discipline in ankle surgery. Dr John Stienstra was the course chairman at the time.

The whole world of foot and ankle surgery has recently seen a resurgence of Minimal Incision Surgery (MIS), and this has been an exciting time. I believe arthroscopy was the original form of MIS, and has evolved exponentially from each decade to the next. Ligament repairs and joint fusions of the ankle are now routinely performed arthroscopically. There is an increasing amount of procedures discussed not only for intra-articular management but also for extra-articular indications. This has quickly expanded outside of the ankle joint to almost every area of the foot. The trend of minimal incisions coupled with expanding fields of view continues to provide newer options for surgeons. We have seen procedures performed endoscopically through plantar fascia and gastrocnemius releases. We are seeing periarticular procedures with Haglund and os trigonum removal, and tendonoscopy procedures are becoming more commonplace. The principles of arthroscopy are now seen in tendon microdebridement procedures, with a debridement wand and ultrasound visualization.

Dr Larry Rubin has always been a leader in the area of foot and ankle arthroscopy. His insight on this advancing area has provided a comprehensive issue with cutting-edge topics and respected authors. The indications will only continue to expand as

Clin Podiatr Med Surg 40 (2023) xiii–xiv
https://doi.org/10.1016/j.cpm.2023.04.001
0891-8422/23/© 2023 Published by Elsevier Inc.

podiatric.theclinics.com

we embrace MIS techniques within the foot and ankle. It is an intriguing time within our profession.

I hope you enjoy this issue.

Thomas J. Chang, DPM
Sonoma County Orthopedic/
Podiatric Specialists
3536 Mendocino Avenue, Suite 300B
Santa Rosa, CA 95403, USA

E-mail address:
thomaschang14@comcast.net

Preface

Foot and Ankle Arthroscopy

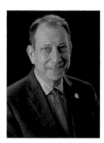

Laurence Rubin, DPM, FACFAS
Editor

It has been 12 years since I was the guest editor for Foot and Ankle Arthroscopy, in *Clinics in Podiatric Medicine and Surgery*. I have been involved with the American College of Foot and Ankle Surgeons (ACFAS) Arthroscopy course for over 25 years and coauthored the ACFAS Arthroscopy e-book with Richard Derner. We continue to improve our skills while progressing our field. The articles in this issue are very different than they were 12 years ago. This demonstrates how far we truly have come. I don't believe that I would have ever considered using arthroscopy for total ankle replacement (TAR), trauma, or ankle instability when I did the last *Clinics in Podiatric Medicine and Surgery*.

I have asked, what I personally consider, the best arthroscopic surgeons in our field to share their experience and expertise with the reader. They have done a masterful job in covering the material. I want to thank them all for their contributions to this issue and to the field of arthroscopic Foot and Ankle Surgery.

To the reader, this is the perfect reference when considering an arthroscopic surgery that is not basic or traditional. The authors have done a great job of providing you the basics of those unique procedures.

As always, I must give a shout out to my mentors in arthroscopy: Harold Vogler and John Stienstra. I know a thank you is not enough, but nothing could be enough—Thank you!!!

I would like to dedicate this *Clinics in Podiatric Medicine and Surgery* to my family: my sons and daughters-in-law: Sam, Tucker, Rachel, and Hallie; my grandson, Harrison;

Clin Podiatr Med Surg 40 (2023) xv–xvi
https://doi.org/10.1016/j.cpm.2023.03.006
0891-8422/23/© 2023 Published by Elsevier Inc.

podiatric.theclinics.com

and especially, my wife, Nancy. Thank you for allowing even more time to devote to my profession!

Laurence Rubin, DPM, FACFAS
Foot and Ankle Surgical Fellowship of Virginia
7016 Lee Park Road, Suite 105
Mechanicsville, VA 23111, USA

E-mail address:
Lgrubin1413@gmail.com

Soft Tissue Pathology

Amber M. Shane, DPM, FACFAS[a,b,*],
Christopher L. Reeves, DPM, FACFAS[b,c], Garrett B. Nguyen, DPM[b],
Thomas D. Ferrise, DPM[b], Phillip M. Calaj, DPM[b]

KEYWORDS

- Soft tissue pathology • Posttraumatic lesions • Posttraumatic adhesions
- Ankle impingement lesions • Syndesmotic impingement • Arthrofibrosis
- Inflammatory synovitis • Crystalline synovitis • Infectious synovitis
- Hemophilic arthropathy • Degenerative synovitis • Congenital plicae
- Neoplastic disorders • Pigmented villonodular synovitis • Synovial chondromatosis

KEY POINTS

- A variety of pathologies can lead to soft tissue abnormalities within the ankle joint.
- They are often chronic in nature and involve synovial or fibrocartilaginous tissue.
- In general, the etiology of ankle soft tissue disorders can be classified as traumatic, inflammatory, and congenital/neoplastic.
- Performing an arthroscopy of the joint can confirm the diagnosis and enable decisive therapy if the surgeon has a strong suspicion that intraarticular soft tissue disease is present.
- The goal of diagnosing and treating soft tissue pathologies of the ankle is to restore anatomic and physiologic motion, reduce pain, optimize functional return to activity, and decrease the chance of recurrence while minimizing complications.

INTRODUCTION

A broad range of diseases can lead to soft tissue abnormalities within the ankle joint. They are often chronic in nature and involve synovial or fibrocartilaginous tissue.[1] Patients frequently complain of ongoing discomfort, edema, and functional difficulties. Many of these disorders can develop into irreversible joint degeneration if left untreated. Fortunately, once recognized, they frequently respond favorably to available therapies, with arthroscopic debridement playing a significant role.

[a] Department of Podiatric Surgery Advent Health System, Advent Health East Orlando Podiatric Surgery Residency, Upperline Health, 250 North Alafaya Trail Suite 1115, Orlando, FL 32828, USA; [b] Department of Podiatric Surgery, Advent Health East Orlando Podiatric Surgery Residency, 250 North Alafaya Trail Suite 1115, Orlando, FL 32828, USA; [c] Rothman Institute, Foot and Ankle Surgery, Advent Health East Orlando Hospital, 7727 Lake Underhill Road, Orlando, FL 32822, USA
* Corresponding author.
E-mail address: Ashane@upperlinehealth.com

Clin Podiatr Med Surg 40 (2023) 381–395
https://doi.org/10.1016/j.cpm.2023.02.003
0891-8422/23/© 2023 Elsevier Inc. All rights reserved.

podiatric.theclinics.com

The first arthroscopic treatments were carried out on cadaveric knee specimens by Takagi in 1918.[2] At the time, it was believed that the huge size of the cystoscopes, which were 7.3 mm in diameter, prevented foot and ankle arthroscopy. Burman used a 3.5 mm arthroscope to perform the first ankle arthroscopy in 1931, but he felt that the joint's small joint space did not lend itself well to arthroscopic methods.[3] Takagi is credited with creating the methods and typical portals used today after demonstrating great outcomes in his series of ankle arthroscopies in 1939.[2]

Rearfoot and ankle arthroscopy is now widespread, and new methods and treatments are constantly being developed. Arthroscopy is frequently used to treat soft tissue conditions such as instability, synovitis, impingement, arthrofibrosis, and other inflammatory disorders in the rearfoot and ankle. The ability to analyze and treat small joints with minimal stress and quick recovery is now possible because of the development of small-joint arthroscopic technology and better diagnostic investigations. A thorough history and physical examination should serve as the basis for evaluation, which should then be followed by any necessary clinical, laboratory, and imaging tests. In general, the etiology of ankle soft tissue disorders can be classified as traumatic, inflammatory, and congenital/neoplastic. The main goal of this article is to identify arthroscopic soft tissue ankle pathology and discuss potential treatment options.

POSTTRAUMATIC LESIONS

In the US, there are about 1 million acute ankle injuries every year, with lateral ankle sprains accounting for the great majority of these cases.[4] Ankle sprains occur frequently in both sports and daily activities, making them a very common injury. 25% of volleyball injuries, 45% of basketball injuries, and 31% of soccer injuries are attributed to ankle sprains.[5] 40% to 50% of individuals with moderate to severe ankle sprains experience chronic problems.[6,7] Localized synovitis and the development of fibrous scar tissue can develop following these injuries.[6,7] Motion of the ankle may result in impingement by the talus or distal tibia when there is a localized synovial or hyalinized fibrocartilaginous scar response. Chronic impingement may lead to the development of fibrocartilage or further synovial hypertrophy. These can cause pain, restrict motion, and ultimately lead to anterior and posterior impingement lesions (Chapters 2 and 3).

The severity of the damage and the tissue's response will determine whether there will be any sequelae, which may range from brief inflammation to long-term pain and discomfort. Other common traumatic soft-tissue pathologies include secondary impingement lesions consisting of Wolin lesions and Basset lesions as well as other nonspecific arthrofibrosis and adhesions.

Syndesmotic Impingement

Injury to the syndesmosis occurs more frequently than is typically acknowledged. When the deltoid ligament is additionally injured, allowing for the displacement of the talus in the mortise, severe syndesmotic disruptions are typically seen. Without obvious clinical instability, however, modest syndesmotic lesions can cause chronic intraarticular ankle discomfort. For all ankle sprains, syndesmotic injuries should be suspected and investigated. Particularly when the mechanism of damage involves external rotation or hyperdorsiflexion, they should be taken into account.[8,9] Syndesmotic injuries are more common among wrestlers, soccer players, and skiers due to their rotational injuries.[10] The use of arthroscopy has improved knowledge of the occurrence of these lesions and can help guide treatment.

Anterolateral or posterolateral soft tissue impingement may be mimicked by a lesion originating from the distal tibiofibular joint and entering the articular space. Pain with weight-bearing activity and range of motion of the ankle joint is the main complaint, precipitated mainly with walking. Patients may describe the pain as a catching or locking sensation secondary to a mass effect within the ankle joint.

These patients often exhibit localized discomfort across the distal portion of the anterior syndesmosis during a physical examination. The squeeze test and external rotation test are typically positive when looking for acute syndesmosis disruption or instability. However, in chronic cases, stress examination may not reveal pain or discomfort. It is vital to take chronic syndesmotic instability into account when considering surgery for a patient with syndesmotic impingement.

Plain radiographs and advanced imaging may help rule out other soft tissue pathologies or osseous lesions. Intraoperative stress examination with fluoroscopy may be utilized to detect syndesmotic laxity if advanced imaging fails to confirm syndesmotic impingement/instability. A mortise view is obtained with the foot internally rotated, followed by a comparable mortise view with the foot forcibly rotated externally. Once syndesmotic impingement is confirmed arthroscopically, a thorough debridement can be performed (**Fig. 1**). Transsyndemostic stabilization can then be addressed if significant widening is observed. Usage of a 3 mm spherical probe or 3.5 mm shaver into the syndesmotic recess during external rotation can indicate a high likelihood of rupture of both the anterior inferior tibiofibular ligament (AITFL) and the interosseous ligament (IOL).[11]

Wolin lesions

Wolin and colleagues[12] published the first description of a mass of hyalinized connective tissue emerging from the anteroinferior aspect of the ankle joint in 1950. A dense mass of white, fibrocartilaginous tissue was discovered during arthrotomy in their investigation of 9 patients with chronic anterolateral ankle joint discomfort and swelling due to inversion injuries. According to Wolin, the lesion was caused by the inadequate resorption of posttraumatic tissue, for which the shear pressures between the talus and the fibula compressed the scar tissue into a mass. He classified the

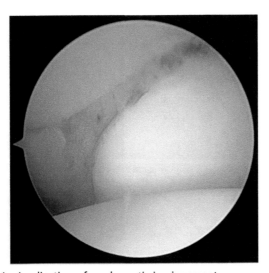

Fig. 1. Arthroscopic visualization of syndesmotic impingement.

lesion as a meniscoid since its appearance resembled that of a meniscus and aptly named it a Wolins lesion. Some authors have, however, questioned the etiology proposing that the lesion is a result of a tear of the anterior talofibular ligament.[13]

A fibrocartilaginous scar may occur in the anterolateral corner of the ankle joint as a result of injury to the anterior talofibular ligament and inferior band of the anterior tibiofibular ligament. These injuries can cause hemarthrosis, which can lead to fibrous tissue hypertrophy in the fibroblastic response. Hemarthrosis can also cause synovitis, which can persist for a long time. Ultimately, the synovitis reorganizes into a well-differentiated meniscoid lesion causing impingement (**Fig. 2**).

On physical examination, patients often report diffuse chronic anterolateral pain and edema with direct palpation. The anterolateral joint line where the fibula is compressed against the talus should be the area of greatest tenderness; nevertheless, these lesions might occasionally be asymptomatic. Upon range of motion, clicking or popping may be present. History and physical examination are mostly used to make the diagnosis, but advanced imaging can be useful in excluding other pathology.

Magnetic resonance imaging (MRI) or computed tomography (CT) with contrast may be beneficial in guiding treatment; however, cost/benefit analysis must be weighed to determine usefulness (**Fig. 3**). Radiographic imaging may provide evidence of an old inversion injury thereby possibly confirming the etiology. In conjunction, intraarticular joint injection can be both therapeutic and diagnostic.

Typically, surgical treatment is warranted to remove the organized meniscoid lesion. Conservative treatment is unlikely to succeed in removing the discomfort. Postoperatively, patients often display a significant improvement in pain and discomfort once the meniscoid lesion is arthroscopically removed from the anterolateral gutter.

Basset lesions

Soft tissue impingements can also be caused by anatomic variations within the anterolateral ankle joint. The accessory fascicle of the anterior inferior talofibular ligament (AITFL) was first identified by Bassett and colleagues[14] as the source of ligamentous impingement in the anterior ankle joint. This anatomic variant is oriented parallel to the main ligament but is separated by a fibrofatty septum, seen in anywhere between 21%

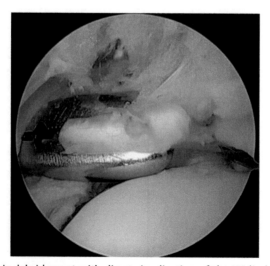

Fig. 2. Arthroscopic debridement with direct visualization of the Wolin lesion.

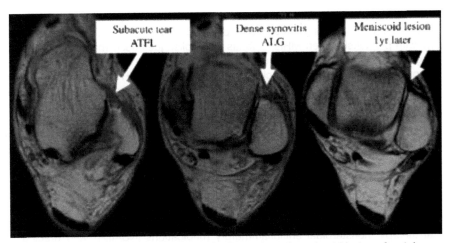

Fig. 3. MRI with 1 year follow-up noting the formation of meniscoid lesion after injury.

and 92% of individuals.[15] The fascicle is observed to attach at the anterolateral corner of the distal tibia and inserts just proximal to the anterior talofibular ligament[16] **(Fig. 4A)**.

Disruption or injury to the accessory fascicle, which is frequently asymptomatic, can stimulate hypertrophic growth and pathology. In the case of inversion ankle sprains, attenuation and laxity of the lateral collateral ligaments can allow for the anterior translation of the talar dome with active or passive dorsiflexion. The inferior aspect of the hypertrophic accessory fascicle often becomes entrapped within the distal tibiofibular recess and the talus. Therefore, pain and discomfort are generated rather by the aberrant position and entrapment of normal anatomic variation than by the presence alone.

Patients with chronic ankle discomfort about the anterolateral region of the ankle following an inversion injury who have a stable ankle and normal plain radiographs should be evaluated for a Bassett lesion. Tenderness will be elicited along the AITFL and dorsolateral talar dome. Additionally, compared to other impingement lesions, the Bassett lesion has been found to occur more frequently and with an audible pop and pain worsening with dorsiflexion and eversion.[14] A thorough assessment must be investigated to further discern between synovial impingement from AITFL entrapment.

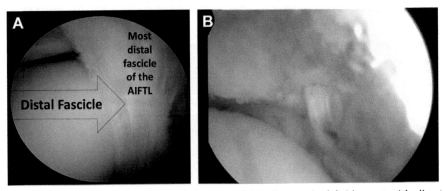

Fig. 4. (A) Accessory distal fascicle of the AITFL (B) Arthroscopic debridement with direct visualization of the Basset lesion.

As with other soft tissue pathologies, advanced imaging may play a role in confirming the diagnosis. To compare arthroscopically confirmed Bassett's ligament pathology with previously taken MRIs, Subhas and colleagues used magnetic resonance imaging data retrospectively to evaluate the presence and reliability. In this, they discovered that 89% of their specimens had an accessory AITFL ligament.[17] Furthermore, Robinson and colleagues[18] concluded that arthrography is a useful tool in the diagnostic toolbox after reporting 100% success with the use of arthrography techniques when examining the AITFL in normal and nonpathologic ankles. The diagnostic value of CT imaging may be limited only to rule out fractures or other osseous pathology.

Conservative treatment may be attempted, incorporating injections, physical therapy for strengthening and flexibility, proprioceptive training, and lateral ankle restabilization. If the recurrence of symptomatic ankle pain is not resolved, surgical intervention is warranted. Akseki and colleagues[19] evaluated 21 patients with symptomatic Basset lesions utilizing conservative treatment options which included physical therapy, nonsteroidal antiinflammatory medications (NSAIDs), and bracing for three months. All 21 patients failed conservative therapy. Contrarily, arthroscopic excision of the thickened and pathologic ligament was helpful in reducing pain without leading to any extra joint instability[20,21] (**Fig. 4**B). Documented improvements have been noted with patients undergoing surgical invention with less than 2 years of ankle joint pain for anterior ankle joint impingement.[21] Thus demonstrating the importance of early diagnosis and excision in achieving positive results.

Arthrofibrosis/Posttraumatic Adhesions

After a fracture or during surgery, arthrofibrosis and posttraumatic adhesions may develop. When a distal fibula fracture or medial malleolus fracture or a mild to moderate ankle sprain results in adhesions, arthroscopy is helpful in removing them. These injuries often cause intraarticular blood to leak into the surrounding tissue causing hemarthrosis. Hemarthrosis that is not aspirated and subsequently absorbed by the synovial joint can cause a significant inflammatory cellular response, fibrous tissue reaction, hyalinization, and eventually chronic synovitis with adhesion (**Fig. 5**A–C). Elevation of proinflammatory cytokines following intraarticular fracture has been shown to increase synovial catabolism and cartilage degradation.[22]

The symptoms are frequently nonspecific and less regional than those reported by the other soft tissue pathologies. On physical examination, diffuse edema and varying degrees of pain are frequently observed. Motion is often slightly restricted with pain upon a range of motion. In severe cases, crepitus can be felt within the ankle joint.

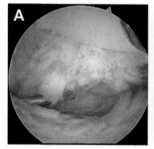 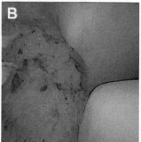 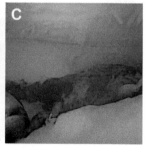

Fig. 5. (A) Subacute fibrous tissue reaction and synovitis (B) Inflamed hypertrophic synovium following acute ankle fracture (C) Hemarthrosis following acute ankle fracture.

Plain radiographs will usually be negative unless significant heterotopic ossifications or other concomitant bony pathology is present. MRI may help evaluate the extent of the adhesion or arthrosis, but this is often equivocal. Diagnostic injections should provide significant relief and should be vital in determining whether to proceed with surgical intervention.

Initial treatment should involve conservative care with immobilization, physical therapy, nonsteroidal antiinflammatory, and corticosteroid injections. Should conservative therapy fail, arthroscopic treatment may be warranted. Ferkel and colleagues[23] found good to excellent results following limited arthroscopic synovectomies on 26/31 patients. Numerous fibrous bands or intraarticular adhesions are frequently visible at the time of surgery (**Fig. 6**). Small, insignificant tissue filaments, broad tissue bands, and severe adhesions with concurrent capsulitis are all possible types of adhesions. Joint space narrowing may complicate arthroscopic debridements. To prevent further harm to the already fragile articular cartilage, extreme caution must be exercised.

INFLAMMATORY DISORDERS/SYNOVITIS
Rheumatoid Arthritis

Rheumatoid arthritis (RA) is a chronic systemic disorder of the immune system. The inflammatory disease may affect the foot and ankle in as many as 70–90% of the RA population, unfortunately this increases the risk for structural joint damage.[24] These lower extremity issues may present in early as well as later stages of RA thus it is important to monitor patients with RA closely, early treatment with new and effective medication lowers the need for surgical intervention.[25]

In relation to arthroscopy of the ankle joint in patients with rheumatoid arthritis, synovial villi will appear larger, club like, pale, and edematous.[26] The synovium will often present hyperemic, alongside loose cartilaginous debris in the later stages of the disease.[27] Treatment options vary for ankle joint pain associated to the Rheumatoid Arthritis, typically early treatment options include disease-modifying antirheumatic drugs followed by interleukin-1 receptor or tumor necrosis factor antagonist; however, persistent synovitis has been treated arthroscopically in the wrist, elbow, knee, and now the ankle. Patients with rheumatoid arthritis who undergo arthroscopic

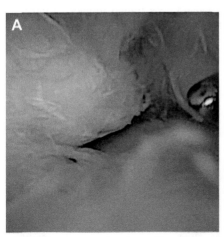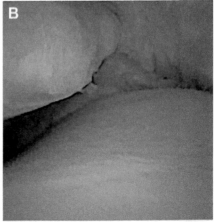

Fig. 6. (*A*) Intraarticular tissue filaments and adhesions (*B*) Status-post ankle joint arthroscopic debridement.

synovectomy of the ankle improved overall when compared to the preop assessment. Early synovectomy in patients with Larsen grades 0 to 1 when compared to grades 2 or 3 leads to better overall results[28]

Crystalline Synovitis

Gout or Pseudogout is inflammatory crystal-induced arthropathies that present with progressive stiffness, persistent aching, rubor, and calor.[29] Gout is caused by monosodium urate monohydrate crystals while pseudo gout is caused by calcium pyrophosphate crystals. Treatment options include anti-inflammatory medications alongside urate-lowering agents if necessary; however, if the arthropathy is recalcitrant, open and arthroscopic surgical options are warranted.[29] Arthroscopy is helpful for both the diagnosis and improvement and clinical symptoms of ankle gouty arthritis. Ankle swelling, pain, function, and the mean acute gouty attacks decreased significantly.[30] Arthroscopic resection of tophi can minimize postoperative wounds, and increase the speed of recovery[31] (**Fig. 7**).

Infectious Synovitis

Septic arthrosis while rare is a serious infection that may lead to cartilage erosion, synovitis, and possibly osteomyelitis.[32] Serum and joint fluid analysis typically demonstrate Staphylococcus Aureus, treatment typically requires surgical drainage and intravenous antibiotic therapy.[33] Arthroscopic synovectomy, irrigation, and debridement presents similar outcomes to the traditional approach with fewer complications. Infections classified up to Gachter stage III which consists of a thickened synovial membrane, compartment formation, with no radiological alterations can be arthroscopically treated.[34]

Hemophilic Arthropathy

Hemophilia is a hereditary hemorrhagic disorder where prolonged bleeding is present with or without trauma.[35] Recurrent hemorrhage often found in the knee and ankle joints leads to synovial hypertrophy and hemosiderin deposition, fibrosis, OCD, and subchondral damage.[36,37] Repetitive synovitis leads to continual joint destruction to the point of possible ankylosis due to the cytokines released.[38] Arthroscopic treatment options vary depending on the level of arthropathy and this includes, debridement/synovectomy, bone marrow-derived cells transplantation, arthrodesis, and arthroplasty, this is a good option for hemophiliacs as fewer clotting factors are needed postoperatively; however, it is important to consider radioactive synovectomy.[39,40]

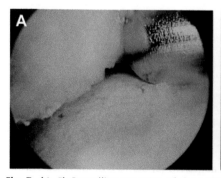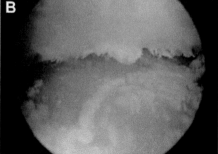

Fig. 7. (*A, B*) Crystalline synovitis of the ankle joint.

MISCELLANEOUS DISORDERS
Congenital Plicae

Plicae, also known as synovial bands, are described as folds within the synovium of a joint. Thus, they can occur in any synovial joint, most commonly described in the knee.[41] Congenital plica are commonly unintentional discoveries made during arthroscopic inspection. Although the exact cause of ankle plica remains unclear, one described cause of the knee is likely due to be an embryological remnant of the mesenchymal tissue during development.[42] These asymptomatic plica may become symptomatic by repetitive or single traumatic events. Symptomatic plica is associated with clicking, popping, and pain with joint motion. With the use of arthroscopy, the frequency of symptomatic plica has become more common. Symptomatic as well as congenital asymptomatic plica have been arthroscopically debrided with favorable outcomes.[43,44]

Neoplastic Disorders

Although rare, there remain many neoplastic disorders of the foot and ankle. A multidisciplinary approach is advised when dealing with this complex pathology. Complete resection with clear histologic margins remains the gold standard of surgical intervention.[45] Many soft tissue neoplasms of the ankle are amenable to arthroscopic resection. Tenosynovial giant cell tumor is a generalized class of neoplasm originating from tendon, synovium, and bursae. These include pigmented villonodular synovitis, more to follow. Even so, standard management of most malignant neoplasms is reported as open procedures.[46]

Pigmented Villonodular Synovitis

Pigmented villonodular synovitis (PVNS) is a subclass of tenosynovial giant cell tumor. Etiology is unclear as an inflammatory process or neoplastic disorder secondary to the locally aggressive but benign nature of the pathology. The recurrence rate after resection is variable and reported between 8% and 60%.[47] Histologic examination is consistent with iron deposition, inflammation, hylanization, and fibrosis with the presence of giant cells.[48] Clinically the patient may present with decreased ankle range of motion, pain with weightbearing, and joint effusion.

PVNS can be divided into 2 subclasses localized and diffuse PVNS. Localized PVNS (LPVNS) is a solitary pedunculated lesion with surrounding tissue absent of disease, and less aggressive. Diffuse PVNS (DPVNS) is a locally more aggressive form that encomopasses the entirety of a synovial space, most commonly a synovial joint (**Fig. 8**). LPVNS is more common than DPVNS. Arthroscopic debridement is a viable diagnostic and treatment option for LPVNS.[49] DPVNS is more commonly treated with open arthrotomy.

Synovial Chondromatosis

Synovial chondromatosis is a rare progressive soft tissue-initiated disease of synovial joints. Identified by cartilaginous nodules formed within the synovial tissue of the joint(**Fig. 9A**). It is characterized as a neoplastic disorder due to the progressive metaplastic nature of the disease along with the history of recurrence. Recurrence and progression can result in chondrosarcoma in approximately 5% of cases.[50] Generally this condition is described in 3 stages classified by Milgram. Stage one: Active intrasynovial disease without loose bodies. Stage 2: Transitional lesions with both active intrasynovial proliferation and free loose bodies. Stage 3: Multiple free osteochondral bodies without intrasynovial disease.[51]

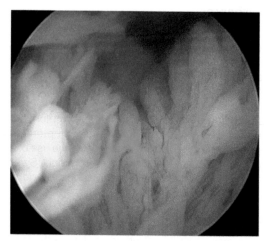

Fig. 8. Pigmented villonodular synovitis of the ankle joint.

Clinical manifestations are stage dependent and for the most part, nonspecific. Joint locking, clicking, and effusion can be appreciated clinically. Pain is elicited with both weight-bearing and nonweight bearing. Intuitively, symptom intensity and frequency increase with stage progression.

Synovial chondromatosis differs from other loose body-inducing pathologies of the ankle such as osteochondritis dissecans, osteoarthritis, and fracture in that it is initiated by the synovial tissue rather than bone. Treatment is dependent upon the stage of the disease. Stage 1 is generally treated conservatively. Stages 2 and 3 are treated with open synovectomy and removal of all foreign bodies with a recurrence rate of 12%.[52] However as arthroscopic techniques and technologies become more advanced, arthroscopic debridement is also a viable alternative(**Fig. 9**B). One systematic review showed a low complication rate. Recurrence was only seen in one patient (5%), which was nonprogressive, likely secondary to incomplete debridement.[53] Arthroscopy does have a place in Stage 1 for diagnostic purposes and direct visualization for accurate biopsy.

ARTHROSCOPIC TREATMENT OF SOFT TISSUE PATHOLOGY
Surgical Technique

Arthroscopic debridement for the treatment of the above-mentioned diseases has a similar approach and technique. As with any surgical skill, arthroscopy needs to be built on a foundation of simplicity before attempting more technically challenging cases. The authors suggest beginning with a synovectomy and diagnostic purposes prior to attempting more complex pathology with limited visibility and maneuverability. Anterior approach is initiated by the identification of topographical anatomy. The medial aspect of the anterior tibial tendon, medial malleolus, joint line, superficial peroneal nerve (SPN), and lateral malleolus are identified. Tracing the SPN can be done by flexing the fourth digit without the overhead operating room lights on the field and prior to the use of tourniquet and exsanguination Placement of the anteromedial portal is accomplished using an 18 gauge spinal needle on a 20cc syringe. Pierce the joint just medial to the tibialis anterior tendon to avoid lacerating the saphenous vein. The authors prefer lactated ringers with epinephrine for fluid management. Approximately 15cc of fluid is utilized to insufflate the joint. Proper intraarticular placement

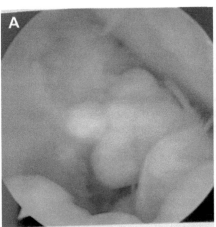 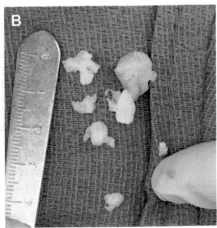

Fig. 9. (A, B) Synovial chondromatosis of the ankle joint.

of the needle can be confirmed by lightly palpating the lateral aspect of the ankle joint for bulging joint capsule. Then a #11 blade is utilized to make a superficial dissection in line with the previous spinal needle. A straight hemostat is used at an oblique angle laterally to palpate joint capsule before bluntly penetrating the joint, proper location will be confirmed with the expulsion of the injected fluid. A blunt trochar is utilized to place the medial portal and the 2.7 mm arthroscope is introduced. Pressure-sensitive ingress is placed between 30 and 40 mmhg. A preliminary inspection of the joint is performed as the 18 gauge spinal needle is placed lateral to the SPN and medial to the medial malleolus. This confirms the location of the lateral portal and is entered in a similar fashion to the medial portal. The working portal and the viewing portal can be switched as needed to better access the necessary pathology.

Advances in technology have assisted the arthroscopist in the treatment of these complex pathologies. The standard 2.7 mm and 4.0 mm arthroscope is now accompanied by a smaller 1.7 mm scope which makes maneuvering throughout the joint more accessible and forgiving while simplifying fluid management. Microshavers have customized torque settings as well as RPM. Thicker more robust tissue can easily be debrided by adjusting the torque setting with increased suction. . Additionally, the use of an ablation/RF wand allows for the "shrinking" of pathologic tissue. Through the use of electrolyte plasmarization, the soft tissue is destroyed. Side effects of this new technique of debridement are over aggressive debridement leading to the debridement of the fibrous capsule and possibly into the anterior neurovascular bundle. The ablation wand also subsequently does heat the surrounding fluid and can decorticate bone. The authors regularly use the ablation/RF wand to increase the working space around the camera entry to increase visualization during the preliminary joint inspection.

SUMMARY

From acute and self-limited to chronic and crippling, the spectrum of pathology that can affect the intraarticular soft tissues of the ankle joint is wide. Even though many of these disorders have some connection to trauma, the specific pathophysiology can be multifactorial and include inflammatory disorders as well as congenital/neoplastic disorders. An analytic technique should be used to pursue the diagnosis.

The most important components of the work-up are often a thorough history and physical examination, closely followed by a solid comprehension of the potential disease processes that may manifest in this anatomic region. It is impossible to overestimate the importance of a diagnostic anesthetic injection for identifying intraarticular disease because it is a quick and uncomplicated approach with a high yield. Imaging tests such as plain radiographs, MRI, and CT scans can be helpful in determining the existence and severity of certain pathologies or excluding other sources of symptoms. Performing an arthroscopy of the joint can confirm the diagnosis and enable decisive therapy if the surgeon has a strong suspicion that intraarticular soft tissue disease is present.

The severity of the symptoms and the duration of the pathology will dictate treatment options. With minor symptoms or pathologies with a low likelihood of joint degradation, conservative therapeutic methods include activity modification, NSAIDs, physical therapy, and corticosteroid administration may be indicated. To avoid undesirable results that could result from waiting, surgical correction may need to be pursued sooner in some circumstances. In the end, the goal of diagnosing and treating soft tissue pathologies of the ankle is to restore anatomic and physiologic motion, reduce pain, optimize functional return to activity, and decrease the chance of recurrence while minimizing complications. When encountering such pathology, surgeons should always rely on their own judgment and experience.

CLINICS CARE POINTS

- With acute trauma, arthroscopic debridement of hemarthrosis can decrease the inflammatory response and prevent adhesions, synovial catabolism, and cartilage degradation.
- Impingement lesions, whether posttraumatic or anatomic, should be evaluated with a thorough history and physical; arthroscopic debridement is often warranted as conservative therapy is unlikely to succeed.
- When treating recalcitrant Rheumatoid arthritis, persistent synovitis can be treated arthroscopically.
- Consider lowering complications for infectious synovitis treatment with an arthroscopic approach.
- When monitoring hemophiliacs for prolonged bleeding, consider a treatment that requires fewer clotting factors postoperatively.
- When attempting to diagnose possible crystalline synovitis, consider using arthroscopy as a diagnostic tool.
- Synovial chondromatosis can be treated with extensive synovial debridement, however, avoid under debridement as recurrence can lead to metaplasia.
- When encountering congenital plica, synovial bands, or folds; aggressive debridement should be performed as it has shown favorable outcomes without increased complication rates.
- Understanding of neurovascular anatomy is imperative when the debridement of synovial/soft tissue disorders is required to avoid catastrophic compromise intraoperatively.

DISCLOSURE

Authors have nothing to disclose.

REFERENCES

1. Boynton MD, Guhl JF. Soft tissue pathology. Foot and Ankle Arthroscopy 2004;99–114.
2. Takagi K. The arthroscope. J Jpn Orthop Assoc 1939;14:359.
3. Burman MS. Arthroscopy of direct visualization of joints: an experimental cadaver study. J Bone Joint Surg 1931;13:669–74.
4. Wexler RK. The injured ankle. Am Fam Physician 1998;57(3):474.
5. Garrick JG. The frequency of injury, mechanism of injury, and epidemiology of ankle sprains. Am J Sports Med 1977;5:241–2.
6. Freeman M. Instability of the foot after injuries to the lateral ligament of the ankle. J Bone Joint Surg Br 1965;47:669.
7. Smith RW, Reischl SF. Treatment of ankle sprains in young athletes. Am J Sports Med 1986;14:465–71.
8. Edwards GS, DeLee JC. Ankle diastasis without fracture. Foot Ankle 1984;4:305.
9. Hopkinson WJ, St Pierre P, Ryan JB, et al. Syndesmosis sprains of the ankle. Foot Ankle 1990;10:325.
10. Fristchy D. An unusual ankle injury in top skiers. Am J Sports Med 1989;17:282.
11. Guyton GP, Defontes K III, Barr CR, et al. Arthroscopic correlates of subtle syndesmotic injury. Foot Ankle Int 2017;38:502–6.
12. Wolin I. Internal derangement of the talofibular component of the ankle. Surg Gynecol Obstet 1950;91:193–200.
13. Andrews JR, Drez DJ, McGinthy JB. Symposium: arthroscopy of joints other than the knee. Contemp Orthop 1984;9(4):71–100.
14. Bassett FH III, Gates HS III, Billys JB, et al. Talar impingement by the anteroinferior tibiofibular ligament. J Bone Joint Surg Am 1990;72:55–9.
15. Nikolopoulos CE, Tsirikos AI, Sourmelis S, et al. The accessory anteroinferior tibiofibular ligament as a cause of talar impingement: a cadaveric study. Am J Sports Med 2004;32:389–95.
16. Akseki D, Pinar H, Bozkurt M, et al. The distal fascicle of the anterior inferior tibiofibular ligament as a cause of anterolateral ankle impingement. Acta Orthop Scand 1999;70(5):478–82.
17. Subhas N, Vinson EN, Cothran RL, et al. MRI appearance of surgically proven abnormal accessory anterior-inferior tibiofibular ligament (Bassett's ligament). Skeletal Radiol 2008;37:27–33.
18. Robinson P, White LM, Salonen DC, et al. Anterolateral ankle impingement: mr arthrographic assessment of the anterolateral recess. Radiology 2001;221:186–90.
19. Akseki D, Pinar H, Yaldiz K, et al. The anterior inferior tibiofibular ligament and talar impingement: a cadaveric study. Knee Surg Sports Traumatol Arthrosc 2002;10:321–6.
20. Tol JL, Verheyen CP, van Dijk CN. Arthroscopic treatment of anterior impingement in the ankle. J Bone Joint Surg Br 2001;83:9–13.
21. van Dijk CN, Tol JL, Verheyen CC. A prospective study of prognostic factors concerning the outcome of arthroscopic surgery for anterior ankle impingement. Am J Sports Med 1997;26(6):737–45.
22. Pham TM, Frinch LH, Lambertsen KL, et al. Elevation of inflammatory cytokines and proteins after intra-articular ankle fracture: a cross-sectional study of 47 ankle fracture patients. Mediators Inflamm 2021;2021:8897440.
23. Ferkel RD, Karzel RP, Del Pizzo W, et al. Arthroscopic treatment of anterolateral impingement of the ankle. Am J Sports Med 1991;19(5):440–6.

24. Simonsen MB, Hørslev-Petersen K, Cöster MC, et al. Foot and ankle problems in patients with rheumatoid arthritis in 2019: still an important issue. ACR open rheumatol 2021;3(6):396–402.

25. Prevoo ML, van 't Hof MA, Kuper HH, et al. Modified disease activity scores that include twenty-eight-joint counts: development and validation in a prospective longitudinal study of patients with rheumatoid arthritis. Arthritis Rheum 1995; 38:44–8.

26. Chaturvedi V, Thabah MM, Ravindran V, et al. Medical arthroscopy: a tool for diagnosis and research in rheumatology. Int J Rheum Dis 2017;20:145–53.

27. Altman RD, Gray R. Diagnostic and therapeutic uses of the arthroscope in rheumatoid arthritis and osteoarthritis. Am J Med 1983;75:50–5.

28. Choi WJ, Choi GW, Jin WL. Arthroscopic synovectomy of the ankle in rheumatoid arthritis. Arthroscopy 2013;29:133–40.

29. Wang CC, Lien SB, Huang GS, et al. Arthroscopic elimination of monosodium urate deposition of the first metatarsophalangeal joint reduces the recurrence of gout. Arthroscopy 2009;25:153–8.

30. Li HI, Li SY, Qui W, et al. Clinical observation of arthroscopic debridement for acute gouty arthritis of the ankle. Zhongguo Gu Shang 2016;29:258–60.

31. Pan F, Li Q, Tang X, et al. Method and effectiveness of arthroscopic debridement for treating gouty arthritis of the knee. Zhongguo Xiu Fu Chong Jian Wai Ke Za Zhi 2011;25:937–40.

32. Mankovecky MR, Roukis TS. Arthroscopic synovectomy, irrigation, and debridement for treatment of septic ankle arthrosis: a systematic review and case series. J Foot Ankle Surg 2014;53(5):615–9.

33. Movassaghi K, Wakefield C, Bohl DD, et al. Septic arthritis of the native ankle. JBJS Reviews 2019;7(3):e6.

34. Romanò CL, Romanò D, Logoluso N, et al. Bone and joint infections in adults: a comprehensive classification proposal. Eur Orthop Traumatol 2011;1(6):207–17.

35. Mehta P, Reddivari AKR. Hemophilia. Treasure Island (FL): StatPearls Publishing; 2022. Updated 2021 Dec 31]. In: StatPearls [Internet.

36. Ng WH, Chu WC, Shing MK, et al. Role of imaging in management of hemophilic patients. Am J Roentgenol 2005;124(5):1619–23.

37. Gualtierotti R, Solimeno LP, Peyvandi F. Hemophilic arthropathy: current knowledge and future perspectives. J Thromb Haemost 2021;19(9):2112–21.

38. Roosendaal G, Vianen ME, Wenting MJ, et al. Iron deposits and catabolic properties of synovial tissue from patients with haemophilia. J Bone Joint Surg British 1998;80(3):540–5.

39. Tonogai I, Sairyo K. A case of arthroscopic ankle arthrodesis for hemophilic arthropathy of the bilateral ankles. Int J Surg Case Rep 2020;74:251–6.

40. Greco T, Polichetti C, Cannella A, et al. Ankle hemophilic arthropathy: literature review. Am J Blood Res 2021;11(3):206–16.

41. Lee PYF, Nixion A, Chandratreya A, et al. Synovial plica syndrome of the knee: a commonly overlooked cause of anterior knee pain. Surg J 2017;3(1):e9–16.

42. Ogata S, Uhthoff HK. The development of synovial plicae in human knee joints: an embryologic study. Arthroscopy 1990;6(4):315–21.

43. Amendola A, Petrik J, Webster-Bogaert S. Ankle arthroscopy: outcome in 79 consecutive patients. Arthroscopy 1996;12(5):565–73.

44. Beaudet P, van Rooij F, Saffarini M, et al. Intra-articular fibrous bands at the tibiotalar joint: diagnosis and outcomes of arthroscopic removal in 4 ankles. J Exp Orthop 2021;8(1):42.

45. Ring A, Kirchhoff P, Goertz O, et al. Reconstruction of soft-tissue defects at the foot and ankle after oncological resection. Front Surg 2016;3:15.

46. Spierenburg G, Lancaster ST, van der Heijden L, et al. Management of tenosynovial giant cell tumour of the foot and ankle. Bone Joint Lett J 2021;103-B(4):788–94.

47. Sharma V, Cheng EY. Outcomes after excision of pigmented villonodular synovitis of the knee. Clin Orthop Relat Res 2009;467(11):2852–8.

48. Flandry F, Hughston JC, McCann SB, et al. Diagnostic features of diffuse pigmented villonodular synovitis of the knee. Clin Orthop Relat Res 1994;298:212–20.

49. Morelli F, Princi G, Rossato A, et al. Pigmented villonodular synovitis: a rare case of anterior ankle impingement. J Orthop Case Rep 2019;10(1):16–8.

50. Davis RI, Hamilton A, Biggart JD. Primary synovial chondromatosis: a clinicopathologic review and assessment of malignant potential. Hum Pathol 1998;29(7):683–8.

51. Milgram JW. Synovial osteochondromatosis: a histopathological study of thirty cases. J Bone Joint Surg Am 1977;59(6):792–801.

52. Maurice H, Crone M, Watt I. Synovial chondromatosis. J Bone Joint Surg Br 1988;70(5):807–11.

53. Al Farii H, Doyle-Kelly C, Marwan Y, et al. Arthroscopic management of synovial chondromatosis of the ankle joint: a systematic review of the literature. JBJS Rev 2020;8(9):e2000045.

Arthroscopic Treatment of Anterior Ankle Impingement

Michael D. Dujela, DPM, FACFAS*, Brian E. Houng, DPM, MS, AACFAS

KEYWORDS

- Ankle arthroscopy • Ankle osteophyte • Tibiotalar impingement • Ankle arthritis
- Ankle instability

KEY POINTS

- Good to excellent results are obtained in 80% to 90% of patients with arthroscopic reduction of anterior tibiotalar osteophytes.
- It is critical to assess for ankle (medial and lateral) and subtalar joint instability that is often associated with osteophyte formation and may need to be simultaneously addressed.
- Diagnostic blocks provide not only therapeutic value, but also diagnostic information particularly in patients who do not show ankle pathology on advanced imaging.
- Synovial impingement secondary to inflammatory changes is the primary cause of pain.
- Removal of osteophytes related to osteoarthritis has a poor prognosis when compared with patients with healthy underlying cartilage.

INTRODUCTION

Anterior ankle impingement (AAI) is characterized by pain in the anterior aspect of the tibiotalar joint during dorsiflexion and may be associated with limited dorsiflexion range of motion.[1,2] First described in 1942 as "athlete's ankle" and later termed "footballer's ankle" in 1949, AAI was often observed among athletes.[1–5] This syndrome refers to entrapment or abutting of structures in the anterior ankle joint during dorsiflexion that can lead to pain and/or restricted motion. AAI can be divided into bony impingement and soft-tissue impingement and further subdivided by location into anterolateral, anterior, and anteromedial impingement.[1–3] Although the etiologies often overlap, anterolateral impingement is frequently caused by soft-tissue impingement, whereas anteromedial impingement is commonly due to osseous impingement.[3–5] This article reviews the most recent literature on AAI and the etiology, clinical and diagnostic evaluation, operative and nonoperative treatments, and outcomes.

Advanced Reconstructive Foot and Ankle Surgery, Washington Orthopaedic Center, 1900 Cooks Hill Road, Centralia, WA 98532, USA
* Corresponding author.
E-mail address: michaeldujela@yahoo.com

Clin Podiatr Med Surg 40 (2023) 397–411
https://doi.org/10.1016/j.cpm.2022.12.001
0891-8422/23/© 2022 Elsevier Inc. All rights reserved.

podiatric.theclinics.com

Anterior Impingement

The formation of exostoses in the anterior distal tibia and the articulating margin of the dorsal anterior talus is a common example of osseous AAI. Previously thought of as an injury response due to repetitive hyper-plantarflexion and traction on the capsular structures, these bony abnormalities have been found to be intra-articular and within the tibiotalar joint capsular attachments.[6,7] This theory has since been discredited and it is now believed that anterior impingement is due to repetitive dorsiflexion and/or impaction of the anterior ankle joint structures. This results in periosteal hemorrhage, chondral and trabecular injury and subsequent formation of osseous proliferations.[5–7]

Osseous impingement can be classified based on size and location of the exostoses according to the Scranton and McDermott classification, and by degree of osteoarthritis according to the van Dijk classification.[7] The morphology of anterior ankle exostoses has been studied and were previously referred to as "kissing osteophytes." However, computed tomography (CT) scans have shown that tibial exostoses have been found to lie lateral to midline, whereas talar exostoses have been found to be medial. As a result, the exostoses are not abutting against each other with dorsiflexion, but rather, they fit into a trough now referred to as a "tram-track lesion" or "divot sign."[8]

Intra-articular soft tissue in the anterior tibiotalar joint can also contribute to impingement and may be present with or without the presence of osseous exostoses. Synovial and adipose tissue are present in the anterior ankle joint, and these structures can become compressed with dorsiflexion. Limited space in the anterior ankle joint can cause entrapment, which results in chronic inflammation, synovitis, and hypertrophy of capsular structures. Fibrous bands and the distal band of the anterior inferior tibiofibular ligament (AITFL) can also be a source of impingement.[6]

Anteromedial Impingement

Multiples theories exist describing the etiology of anteromedial ankle impingement. Similar to AAI theories, anteromedial impingement theories share the capsular traction theory during forced plantarflexion, recurrent microtrauma to the medial ankle structures, and repetitive dorsiflexion of the ankle joint resulting in exostosis formation.[7–9] Additional theories include supination injuries with a rotational component causing tearing of the anterior tibiotalar ligament, anteromedial joint capsule, and deltoid ligament.[7–12] Anteromedial "meniscoid" lesions can form from reactive synovitis and thickening of the medial joint capsule.[7,8,10] Scarring of the anterior deltoid ligament with or without medial ankle instability is also observed with anteromedial impingement.[8] Lastly, osteochondral injury of the medial talus against the medial malleolus can cause bony proliferation and anteromedial exostoses.[7,8]

Anterolateral Impingement

Inversion ankle sprains are often associated with anterolateral ankle impingement. It is reported that approximately 3% of all ankle sprains result in anterolateral impingement.[5] Ferkel and colleagues first described this impingement as a process that begins with an ankle inversion injury that creates tears in the anterior talofibular ligament (ATFL) and AITFL.[9,13] Repetitive and continued motion to the incompletely healed ligaments lead to chronic inflammation, hypertrophied synovium, and scar tissue. Pain is thought to be the result of the torn and entrapped hypertrophic soft tissues or lateral ankle ligaments.[9,13] The most common and well-described sources of anterolateral impingement include synovitis, meniscoid lesions, and the inferior fascicle of the AITFL (Bassett's ligament).[5]

Synovitis is caused by the inadequate healing after inversion ankle injury and continued repetitive motion. This leads to chronic inflammation and enlargement of the synovium. In contrast, the formation of hemorrhagic synovitis begins by injury or tearing of the joint capsule, which leads to an intra-articular hematoma that is reabsorbed by the synovium. The synovium subsequently becomes hypertrophic and inflamed with an elastic and firmer quality than synovitis.[5,9] In either case, the enlarged synovium becomes impinged in the lateral gutter, causing anterolateral ankle pain.[9]

A meniscoid lesion, first described by Wolin and colleagues in 1950, is a hyalinized soft-tissue mass that acquired its name due to the similarity in appearance to a torn knee meniscus.[14] They are bands of scar tissue from the ATFL that reside in the lateral gutter.[14] Additional studies described synovial tissue, scarred capsule, and theanterior inferior tibiofibular ligament as sources of these meniscoid lesions contributing to anterolateral impingement.[15,16]

The inferior fascicle of the AITFL was identified as a source of anterolateral ankle impingement after ankle inversion injuries by Bassett and colleagues in 1990.[17] Now, also known as Bassett's ligament, it lies inferior and parallel to the AITFL.[5] Anatomically, its measurements range from 17 to 22 mm in length, 1 to 2 mm in thickness, and 3-5 mm in width and borders the anterolateral shoulder of the talus.[18] As a result, anterolateral impingement associated with Bassett's ligament can lead to cartilage damage in 17% to 89% when observed with ankle arthroscopy.[5,17,18] There are five anatomic variations described by Ray and colleagues of the ligament and its relationship to the talus.[18] Additional anatomic studies revealed that the closer the inferior fascicle was to the ATFL, the more often impingement would occur in the lateral gutter.[19]

Clinical Presentation

AAI often presents in the young, athletic population with a history of inversion ankle sprains. Patients may describe a single traumatic incident or multiple ankle sprains that resulted in chronic ankle pain without complete resolution. Symptoms include pain during physical activity and a popping or catching sensation to the ankle joint.

Physical examination may reveal pain on palpation to the anterolateral talus, lateral gutter, inferior tibiofibular articulation, anterior ankle, medial gutter, or anteromedial aspect of the ankle joint. Dorsiflexion, inversion, and eversion of the ankle joint can all elicit pain. Clicking or popping may be audible or palpable and is often associated with AITFL impingement. Malloy's test can be used to assess for synovial hypertrophy and lateral gutter impingement by applying pressure to the anterior lateral gutter and moving the ankle from plantarflexion to maximum dorsiflexion.[20] This test elicits pain by impinging the hypertrophic synovitis between the distal lateral tibia and the neck of the talus and has a 94.8% sensitivity and 88% specificity.[5,20]

Although pain on palpation may correspond to an anatomic location of possible impingement, it is imperative to rule out other causes of anteromedial, anterior, and anterolateral ankle pain including tibialis anterior tendonitis, tibialis posterior tendonitis, osteochondral lesions, peroneal tendonitis, ankle or subtalar joint arthritis, and tarsal coalitions. As a result, diagnostic and imaging studies are critical for proper diagnosis and subsequent treatment.

Diagnostic Imaging

Radiographic evaluation

Weightbearing radiographs of the ankle should be obtained on initial presentation. Anteroposterior and ankle mortise views are important to evaluate for fractures, syndesmotic injury with widening of the ankle mortise, obvious osteochondral defects, or arthritic processes such as osteophytes in the medial or lateral gutters. The lateral ankle view is capable of detecting anterior exostoses of the tibia and talus; however, these views have been shown to only detect 40% and 32% of tibial and talar osteophytes, respectively.[5] Tol and colleagues showed that the oblique anteromedial impingement view was able to detect anteromedial osteophytes with an 85% and 73% sensitivity for tibial and talar osteophytes, respectively.[21–23] This oblique view is performed by having the patient supine on the table with the x-ray beam tilted 45° in the craniocaudal direction, externally rotating the leg 30° with the foot in plantarflexion[2,21,22] (**Fig. 1**).

Magnetic resonance imaging

Although standard radiographs can be helpful to evaluate osseous abnormalities, MRI is essential for evaluating soft-tissue structures.[5,23,24] They can evaluate for soft-tissue impingement as well as rule out other sources of ankle pain including osteochondral lesions, tendonitis, tarsal coalitions, and osteoarthritis. Although studies report sensitivy and specificity for MRI range widely from 39% to 100% and 50% to 100%, respectively, the most recent study by Ferkel and colleagues in 2010 reports a sensitivity of 83.3% and specificity of 78.6%.[22,25] Axial T1-weighted images are particularly helpful in assessing scarring and hypertrophic synovial tissue in the lateral gutter and sagittal T1-weighted images can show scar formation just anterior to the fibula. These T1-weighted images will show low signal intensity where scarring has formed.[5,22,23,26]

Direct magnetic resonance arthrography (MRA) is an MRI that is performed after a specific joint is injected with a solution containing gadolinium. The main indications for MR arthrography are for the evaluation of ligamentous injuries, impingement syndromes, cartilaginous lesions, osteochondral lesions, loose bodies, and synovial joint disorders.[5,23,24,27–29] Although MRA has been found to be 97% accurate with a sensitivity of 96% and specificity of 100% for detecting anterolateral impingement, it is not as commonly used. This is partly due to the invasive nature of the procedure in addition to not being significantly superior in detecting AAI when compared with traditional MRI.[5,23,27]

Computed tomography

CT is useful in evaluating the specific location and dimensions of the exostoses. It is also helpful in detecting loose bodies, ossicles, and the osseous involvement

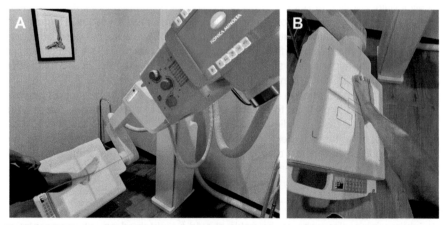

Fig. 1. (A, B) Positioning for an anterior medial impingement view. This oblique view is performed by having the patient positioned supine on the table with the x-ray beam tilted 45° in the craniocaudal direction, externally rotating the leg 30° with the foot in plantarflexion.

associated with osteochondral lesions.[2,5,9,23,24] CT arthrography is a viable option for detecting anterolateral impingement. According to a study by Cochet and colleagues, who showed 97% and 71% sensitivity and specificity, respectively, in diagnosing anterolateral impingement.[26] However, similar to MRA, it is not as favorable due to its invasive nature and does not provide additional value when compared with traditional CT images.

Treatment

Nonoperative management
Conservative treatment often involves rest, ice, anti-inflammatory medications, physical therapy, ankle bracing, shoe modification, or corticosteroid injection. A small heel lift or shoe with elevated heel may reduce anterior impingement symptoms. Physical therapy involves range of motion, proprioceptive, and strengthening exercises. Additional modalities may include ultrasound, electrical stimulation, iontophoresis, and hydrotherapy. After conservative care has been attempted without relief, surgical options can be considered. In patients with longstanding deformity and pain who have obvious mechanical obstruction, consideration may be given to direct surgical treatment.

Diagnostic injection
In many patients, MRI may not show distinct soft-tissue pathology as previously mentioned. The authors' preferred approach is to perform a diagnostic and therapeutic intraarticular injection in all patients who have failed nonoperative therapy and are considering surgery. The patients are evaluated after several minutes to allow the anesthetic component to take effect. At this point, the amount of subjective pain relief is documented. Patients are then seen 3 to 4 weeks post-injection for reassessment. If the pain relief has been substantial and symptoms are mitigated, then nonoperative management is continued. If the pain relief was significant, however short lived, consideration is then given to arthroscopic surgery and the patient is educated about the options including the typical preoperative, perioperative, and postoperative course.

Operative management
Although open and arthroscopic approaches are both viable options and both have good results, studies show that open treatment is associated with higher complication rates. These include wound healing complications, hypertrophic scars, iatrogenic injury to the extensor tendons, and nerve entrapment. Studies also show faster return to activity in the arthroscopic group when compared with open treatment.[1,2]

Historically, ankle arthroscopy was not a common procedure and yielded complication rates of up to 26.4%. However, as techniques and equipment have improved, the complication rates have decreased significantly with reports as low as 3.5%.[13] Most complications are due to nerve or vascular injury, and infection. Currently, ankle arthroscopy is the gold standard for surgical treatment of AAI.[1] The literature supports this recommendation and deems ankle arthroscopy as a safe treatment method.[1,9,13,30–34]

Surgical Technique

Preoperative anatomic marking
The patient is evaluated in the preoperative holding area. Anatomic marking is performed with the patient awake as they are able to actively dorsiflex/invert the ankle to facilitate marking the tibialis anterior tendon that is a key landmark for the anteromedial portal. The anterolateral portal is identified just lateral to the peroneus tertius tendon by dorsiflexing and everting the ankle. Remaining lateral to the peroneus tertius

tendon reduces the risk of injury to the lateral dorsal cutaneous nerve. These maneuvers allow identification of the safe zone in the soft spots at the ankle joint line adjacent to the tendons. It is crucial to develop the portals directly at the level of the joint line. This reduces soft tissue and nerve complications by avoiding overstretching with instrumentation in an attempt to overcome poor visibility.

Patient positioning
The patient is positioned on the operating table specific to the proposed procedure. Various positions are possible depending on anticipated ancillary procedures.

Supine position with a noninvasive distractor
When a distractor is used in a supine position, a well-padded Ferkel leg holder is applied to the proximal thigh. This requires the patient to be placed closer to the head of the bed when the noninvasive distractor is applied so that the distractor has an effective working length. If the patient is too close to the end of the bed, the distractor does not have sufficient working length to achieve adequate traction. A supine position with a noninvasive distractor may be helpful when cartilage work is necessary as in the case of simultaneous management of an osteochondral lesion (**Fig. 2**).

Lateral position with a noninvasive distractor
When an open lateral ankle stabilization is simultaneously performed with arthroscopy of the ankle and osteophyte removal, the author's preference is to place the patient in a lateral position with bean bag support. The leg is externally rotated at the hip and held in position with a leg holder, and a distractor is applied keeping the limb appropriately positioned (**Fig. 3**A, B). The arthroscopy is performed including osteophyte resection and the leg is then removed from the leg holder by the OR personnel maintaining sterility by working under the drapes. The leg is placed on the OR bed supported by a stack of towels in a lateral position and the open lateral ankle stabilization may then be performed.

Supine position without a distractor
The final option is to place the patient supine without the use of a distractor. This is an excellent option in patients who have anterior medial or anterior lateral impingement where partial synovectomy and osteophyte removal is performed and no underlying

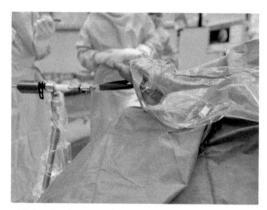

Fig. 2. Limb is placed in a distractor to facilitate access to greater regions of the joint as needed. Care is taken to avoid damage to the anterior neurovascular structures.

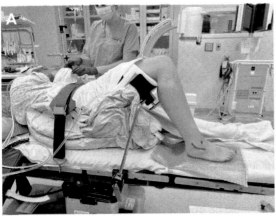
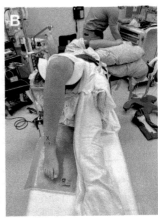

Fig. 3. (A, B) Patient is placed in a lateral decubitus position with beanbag support when combining a lateral ankle stabilization with anterior arthroscopy for removal of tibiotalar osteophytes. The hip is externally rotated and supported with a Ferkel leg holder. Care is taken to appropriately position the patient slightly proximal on the bed to allow sufficient room for working length of the distractor.

cartilage work is necessary. The patient is situated with the heel positioned at the edge of the bed facilitating the ability to dorsiflex the ankle using the surgeon's abdomen. The anterior working space is increased when the ankle is dorsiflexed.

Portal creation
Before creation of the portal, the joint is insufflated with 10 mL of fluid of the surgeon's preference. A 1-cm portal is created medially using a number 11 scalpel blade. Dissection is carried deep with "nick and spread" technique down to the level of the joint where a blunt trocar is introduced obliquely to avoid damage to the articular surface. The foot is placed in a dorsiflexed position during trocar introduction to reduce cartilage injury. It is key to avoid skiving across the anterior soft tissues when introducing this to avoid neurovascular injury. This should be directed slightly off-axis toward the tibia.

Next, a 2.7-mm or 4.0-mm arthroscope is introduced. The author's preference is to use a 4.0 mm arthroscope with a 30° lens which affords a large field of view and does not "crowd" the joint.

A standard arthroscopic evaluation is performed of the anterior compartment of the ankle. This is facilitated with the foot in a dorsiflexed position to take advantage of the anterior working pouch created by the insufflation of 10 mL of fluid. Next, the lateral portal is transilluminated and a spinal needle is introduced lateral to the peroneus tertius tendon under direct visualization.

A 1-cm incision is made and dissection is carried deep with "nick and spread" technique followed by introduction of an obliquely placed blunt trocar again placed carefully to avoid damage to the articular cartilage.

Surgical technique
Once the standard arthroscopic evaluation has been undertaken and pathology noted and documented, surgical repair is undertaken. Initially, any abnormal soft tissue is debrided with a shaver of choice. This is often done through a full radius shaver or

a bone/shaver combo which can range from 3.5 mm to 5.5 mm in size. Clearing any abnormal tissue improves the visualization of cartilage defects or anterior osteophytes.

Anterior osteophyte resection

With the arthroscope inserted through the medial portal, anterior, lateral pathology, and osteophytes are addressed. Conversely, inserting the arthroscope laterally allows visualization of the medial side of the tibia and talus with the burr or bone/shaver combo inserted through the medial portal.

It is important to clear the soft tissues in the space above the osteophytes to improve visibility (**Fig. 4**). This can carefully and safely be done since the soft tissues attach 6 mm proximal to the cartilage rim. Care must be taken to keep the cutting surface of the shaver away from the overlying soft tissues to avoid damage to the neurovascular bundle in the anterior compartment. Damage to the anterior tibial artery is possible (**Fig. 5**). Ideally, the ankle would be dorsiflexed during this maneuver to minimize risk.

With the camera introduced through the medial portal, the lateral portal is the working/functional portal with the introduction of an arthroscopic burr or bone shaver ranging from 4 mm to 5.5 mm in size. A sharp 1/4-inch curved osteotome can also be used but great caution is necessary to avoid cartilage damage. Gentle application of the burr is critical to avoid skipping of the burr and damage to the underlying cartilage (**Fig. 6**).

Distraction of the ankle can be very helpful at this point or alternatively by maximally dorsiflexing the joint to avoid damage to the underlying cartilage as the osteophytes are carefully reduced.

Care is taken to gradually reduce the spur with a bone shaver/burr from proximal to distal and medial to lateral. Anterior medial impingement views are obtained fluoroscopically to confirm adequate reduction of the osteophytes (**Fig. 7**A, B).

Postop management

The patient is non-weight bearing in a posterior splint for the first 10 to 14 days. Depending on the procedure selection, the patient may either be placed in a fracture boot or cast at that point. Early range of motion is encouraged whenever possible to minimize stiffness and adhesions and to promote cartilage health. Partial

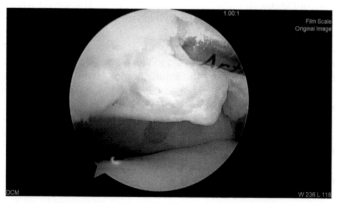

Fig. 4. Soft tissues overlying the anterior tibial osteophyte are carefully removed with a full radius shaver to improve visualization before removal with an arthroscopic burr.

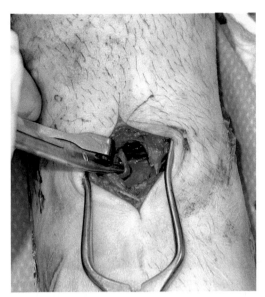

Fig. 5. Care must be taken to avoid damage to the anterior tibial artery that can occur during arthroscopic debridement of anterior tibiotalar osteophytes. Image shows arthrotomy and identification of arterial laceration.

weightbearing may commence as early as 2 weeks; however, with osteochondral lesion treatment this may be delayed until 4 to 6 weeks postop. Physical therapy is initiated as soon as appropriate based on ancillary procedures.

Risks/complications

Although relatively rare, multiple serious complications can occur resulting in long-term disability. When using a distractor, it is important to avoid over tensioning which

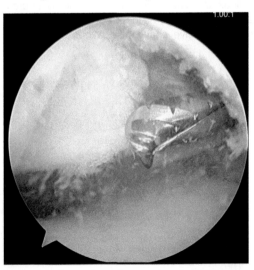

Fig. 6. Arthroscopic burr is used to reduce the anterior distal tibial prominence from distal to proximal and medial to lateral.

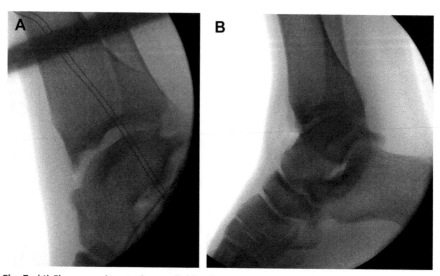

Fig. 7. (*A*) Fluoroscopic anterior medial impingement view is performed intraoperatively to confirm the deformity. (*B*) Fluoroscopic imaging shows removal of the prominent osteophytes from the tibia and talus.

can result in neurologic injury. Consider padding under the dorsal midfoot strap to reduce compression to the deep peroneal nerve under the Guhl distractor strap. Excess fluid ingress particularly while using a pump can result in compartment syndrome. Care should be used to minimize pump pressure, or potentially to use gravity inflow to reduce this risk. In addition, consideration of coban wrap proximal and distal to the joint may theoretically reduce extravasation into the adjacent tissue. Instruments must be handled gently and avoid excess bending forces which could result in breakage and difficult retrieval. Finally, direct vascular or neurologic injury can occur with inadvertent iatrogenic damage via incorrect trocar angle of introduction, improper portal placement or aggressive shaver use. When using a distractor, the anterior

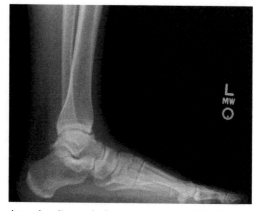

Fig. 8. Preoperative lateral radiograph showing anterior tibiotalar osteophytes.

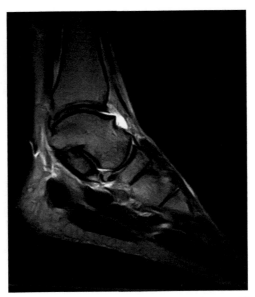

Fig. 9. Sagittal MRI image showing anterior tibiotalar osteophytes with anterior ankle joint effusion and synovitis.

working space is reduced and the potential for injury to the anterior tibial artery and deep peroneal nerve exists.

Case example
A 34-year-old man complained of anterior impingement symptoms that were recalcitrant to nonoperative care. Anterior tibiotalar osteophytes are noted on preoperative lateral radiograph (**Fig. 8**) MRI shows anterior impingement syndrome with joint

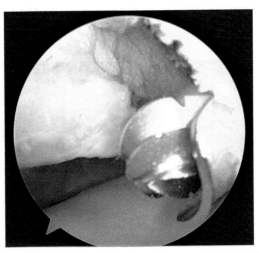

Fig. 10. Arthroscopic view of anterior tibial osteophyte clearly visualized after debridement of synovitis. A 4.0 mm burr is used for resection of the prominence.

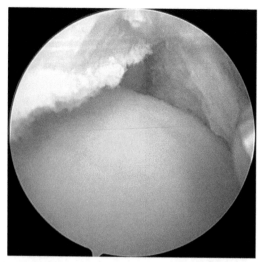

Fig. 11. Arthroscopic view after partial synovectomy and complete resection of osteophytes.

effusion on sagittal image (**Fig. 9**). Arthroscopic partial synovectomy and debridement of osteophytes result in excellent reduction of the prominences and improved range of motion on postoperative lateral charger radiograph (**Figs. 10–12**).

SUMMARY

Arthroscopic reduction of anterior tibiotalar osteophytes is a very efficient and safe procedure that allows early return to function with minimal downtime. The results are reproducible and a high degree of success is demonstrated in the literature. Although the potential for complications exists, the frequency is low with careful attention to detail. Enhanced function and accelerated rehabilitation with early physical therapy are the primary benefits associated with this approach. Patients with minimal

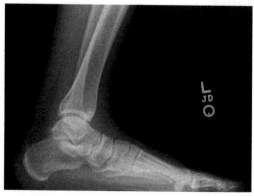

Fig. 12. Lateral radiograph in charger position 4 months' postop showing removal of the osteophytes and improved dorsiflexion.

osteoarthritic changes respond very well to osteophyte reduction and the minimally invasive approach substantially reduces the stiffness and prolonged recovery associated with open arthrotomy.

CLINICS CARE POINTS

- Anterior medial impingement view increases the sensitivity for detecting osteophytes.
- A nonrotated lateral radiographic view may result in missed osteophyte due to greater projection of the anterior lateral tibia
- It is critical to assess for ankle (medial and lateral) and subtalar joint instability which is often associated with osteophyte formation and may need to be simultaneously addressed.
- Diagnostic blocks provide not only therapeutic value, but also diagnostic information particularly in patients who do not show ankle pathology on advanced imaging.
- With care and attention, a noninvasive distractor may be safely used with concomitant osteochondral defects of the talus or tibia exist that are not easily accessible. This minimizes risk to the cartilage during osteophyte resection
- The capsule attaches approximately 6 mm proximal to the joint line, and not to the osteophytes.
- Synovial impingement secondary to inflammatory changes is the primary cause of pain.
- Removal of osteophytes related to osteoarthritis has a poor prognosis when compared with patients with healthy underlying cartilage.

DISCLOSURE

M.D. Dujela: DePuy Synthes, Paragon 28, Sinaptic. B.E. Houng: Nothing to report.

REFERENCES

1. Zwiers R, Wiegerinck JI, Murawski CD, et al. Arthroscopic treatment for anterior ankle impingement: a systematic review of the current literature. Arthroscopy 2015;31(8):1585–96. Epub 2015 Mar 19. PMID: 25801044.
2. Pedro D, Duarte AS, Batista JP, et al. Diagnosis and treatment of anterior ankle impingement: state of the art. J ISAKOS 2020;5(Issue 5):295–303. ISSN 2059-7754.
3. Morris LH. Report of cases of athlete's ankle. J Bone Joint Surg 1943;25:220.
4. McMurray TP. Footballer's ankle. J Bone Joint Surg 1950;32:68–9.
5. Jacobson K, Ng A, Haffner KE. Arthroscopic treatment of anterior ankle impingement. Clin Podiatr Med Surg 2011;28(3):491–510. PMID: 21777781.
6. Lavery KP, McHale KJ, Rossy WH, et al. Ankle impingement. J Orthop Surg Res 2016;11(1):97. PMID: 27608626; PMCID: PMC5016963.
7. Umans H, Cerezal Luiz. Anterior ankle impingement syndromes. Semin Musculoskelet Radiol 2008;12(2):146–53.
8. Murawski CD, Kennedy JG. Anteromedial impingement in the ankle joint: outcomes following arthroscopy. Am J Sports Med 2010;38(10):2017–24.
9. Ross KA, Murawski CD, Smyth NA, et al. Current concepts review: arthroscopic treatment of anterior ankle impingement. Foot Ankle Surg 2017;23(1):1–8. Epub 2016 Feb 15. PMID: 28159036.
10. Egol KA, Parisien JS. Impingement syndrome of the ankle caused by a medial meniscoid lesion. Arthroscopy 1997;13:522–5.

11. Mosier-La Clair SM, Monroe MT, Manoli A, et al. Medial impingement syndrome of the anterior tibiotalar fascicle of the deltoid ligament on the talus. Foot Ankle Int 2000;21:385–91.

12. Robinson P, White LM, Salonen D, et al. Anteromedial impingement of the ankle: using MR arthrography to assess the anteromedial recess. AJR AmJ Roentgenol 2002;78:601–4.

13. Ferkel RD, Karzel RP, Del Pizzo W, et al. Arthroscopic treatment of anterolateral impingement of the ankle. Am J Sports Med 1991;19(5):440–6.

14. Wolin I, Glassman F, Sideman S. Internal derangement of the talofibular component of the ankle. Surg Gynecol Obstet 1950;91:193–200.

15. Schonholtz GJ. Arthroscopic surgery of the shoulder, elbow and ankle. Springfield, IL: Charles C. Thomas; 1986.

16. Keller K, Nasrilari M, Fuller T, et al. The anterior tibio-talar ligament: one reason for anterior ankle impingement. Knee Surg Sports Traumatol Arthrosc 2010;18: 225–32.

17. Bassett FH, Gates HS, Billys JB, et al. Talar impingement by the anteroinferior tibiofibular ligament. A cause of chronic pain in the ankle after inversion sprain. J Bone Joint Surg Am 1990;72:55–9.

18. Ray RG, Kriz BM. Anterior inferior tibiofibular ligament. variations and relationship to the talus. J Am Podiatrmed Assoc 1991;81:479–85.

19. Akseki D, Pinar H, Yaldiz K, et al. The anterior tibiofibular ligament and talar impingement: a cadaveric study. Knee Surg Sports Traumatol Arthrosc 2002; 10:321–6.

20. Molloy S, Solan MC, Bendall SP. Synovial impingement in the ankle. J Bone Joint Surg Br 2003;85(3):330.

21. Tol JL, Verhagen RA, Krips R, et al. The anterior ankle impingement syndrome: diagnostic value of oblique radiographs. Foot Ankle Int 2004;25(2):63–8.

22. Nery C, Baumfeld D. Anterior and posterior ankle impingement syndromes: arthroscopic and endoscopic anatomy and approaches to treatment. Foot Ankle Clin 2021;26(1):155–72. Epub 2020 Sep 9. PMID: 33487238.

23. Berman Z, Tafur M, Ahmed SS, et al. Ankle impingement syndromes: an imaging review. Br J Radiol 2017;90(1070):20160735. Epub 2016 Nov 25. PMID: 27885856; PMCID: PMC5685116.

24. Al-Riyami A, Mohamed Tan HK, Peh WCG. Imaging of ankle impingement syndromes. Can Assoc Radiol J 2017;68(4):431–7.

25. Ferkel RD, Tyorkin M, Applegate GR, et al. MRI evaluation of anterolateral soft tissue impingement of the ankle. Foot Ankle Int 2010;31:655–61.

26. Cochet H, Pele E, Amoretti N, et al. Anterolateral ankle impingement: diagnostic performance of MDCT arthrography and sonography. AJR Am J Roentgenol 2010;194:1575–80.

27. Cerezal L, Llopis E, Canga A, et al. MR arthrography of the ankle: indications and technique. Radiol Clin North Am 2008;46(6):973–94. PMID: 19038607.

28. Tol JL, van Dijk CN. Anterior ankle impingement. Foot Ankle Clin 2006;11(2): 297–310, vi.

29. Parma A, Buda R, Vannini F, et al. Arthroscopic treatment of ankle anterior bony impingement: the long-term clinical outcome. Foot Ankle Int 2014;35(2):148–55.

30. Walsh SJ, Twaddle BC, Rosenfeldt MP, et al. Arthroscopic treatment of anterior ankle impingement: a prospective study of 46 patients with 5-year follow-up. Am J Sports Med 2014;42(11):2722–6.

31. Yang Q, Zhou Y, Xu Y. Arthroscopic debridement of anterior ankle impingement in patients with chronic lateral ankle instability. BMC Musculoskelet Disord 2018; 19(1):239.
32. Barp EA, Erickson JG, Hall JL. Arthroscopic treatment of ankle arthritis. Clin Podiatr Med Surg 2017;34(4):433–44.
33. Katakura M, Odagiri H, Charpail C, et al, Ankle Instability Group. Arthroscopic treatment for anterolateral impingement of the ankle: systematic review and exploration of evidence about role of ankle instability. Orthop Traumatol Surg Res 2021;29:103159. Epub ahead of print. PMID: 34856406.
34. Talusan PG, Toy J, Perez JL, et al. Anterior ankle impingement: diagnosis and treatment. J Am Acad Orthop Surg 2014;22(5):333–9. PMID: 24788449.

Posterior Ankle Impingement

Michael H. Theodoulou, DPM[a,b,]*, Madison Ravine, DPM[c]

KEYWORDS

- Arthroscopy • Endoscopy • Flexor hallucis longus • Os trigonum

KEY POINTS

- Posterior ankle impingement describes a collection of pathologies caused by mechanical compression of the area between the posterior tibia and calcaneus. It is frequently associated with high-level athletic populations.
- Posterior ankle arthroscopy represents an endoscopic approach to an arthroscopic approach, which requires intimate knowledge of the anatomic region due to surrounding neurovascular structures.
- Posterior ankle arthroscopy is a safe and effective treatment of posterior ankle impingement syndrome, allowing for a speedy recovery and quick return to sport compared with open surgical approaches.

INTRODUCTION

Posterior ankle impingement syndrome (PAIS), also known as posterior talar compression syndrome, os trigonum syndrome, posterior ankle block, nutcracker-type impingement, and posterior tibiotalar impingement syndrome, describes a collection of pathologies characterized by compression in the anatomic region between the posterior tibia and calcaneus during plantarflexion.[1,2] The pathologic changes experienced in PAIS result from repeat exposure to constant terminal plantarflexion or local recurrent trauma. Compression may be caused by osseous impingement, such as an os trigonum or prominent posterolateral process, soft-tissue impingement or ligamentous hypertrophies, such as the posterior tibiotalar ligament or the intramalleolar ligament, or a combination thereof.[3] Other causes may include anatomic anomalies, such as low-lying flexor hallucis longus (FHL) muscle belly or aberrant accessory musculature.[4,5] The cause and pathologic anatomic features are heterogenous, and several pathologic conditions can result in PAIS.[5] Athletes are the most commonly affected population by repetitive plantarflexion movements of the foot and ankle,

[a] Podiatric Surgery, Cambridge Health Alliance, Cambridge, MA, USA; [b] Harvard Medical School, 1439 Cambridge Street, Cambridge, MA 02139, USA; [c] Cambridge Health Alliance Podiatric Medicine & Surgery Residency Program, 1439 Cambridge Street, Cambridge, MA 02139, USA
* Corresponding author.
E-mail address: mtheodoulou@challiance.org

Clin Podiatr Med Surg 40 (2023) 413–424
https://doi.org/10.1016/j.cpm.2022.12.002

particularly ballet dancers, soccer players, downhill runners, and football players. Not only does this population present with high physical demand, but it also requires early rehabilitation and prompt return to sport. With the growing advances in arthroscopy, posterior ankle arthroscopy has become an indispensable tool in diagnosing and managing posterior ankle pathology, including PAIS.[6] The aim of this article was to review the pertinent anatomy and pathophysiology of PAIS and to highlight surgical intervention, explicitly using an arthroscopic technique.

PERTINENT ANATOMY

The posterior ankle joint complex is a window well defined by certain anatomic borders. Medially, it is bound by the flexor tendons of the leg, including (from superficial to deep) the posterior tibial tendon, the flexor digitorum longus, and the FHL. The FHL tendon is a critical medial boundary during arthroscopy because the neurovascular bundle lies just medial or posterior to this structure (**Fig. 1**). Laterally, the peroneal tendons are a boundary, protecting the sural nerve and small saphenous vein during arthroscopy. Posteriorly, this window is bound by the Achilles tendon and anteriorly bound by the tibiotalar and talocalcaneal joints. Inferiorly lies the calcaneal tuber. Lying within this defined anatomic vault is adipose tissue, frequently referred to as Kager's triangle.[2,7,8] Posterior ankle arthroscopy has highlighted the need for intimate anatomic knowledge of this window due to the proximity of neurovascular structures.[9]

In 2002, Sitler and colleagues published an anatomic cadaver study evaluating structures at risk when performing posterior ankle arthroscopy through posteromedial and posterolateral portals as described by van Dijk and colleagues in 2000.[10] They used both open dissection and advanced imaging to define the proximity of vital structures to the above portals, placed immediately adjacent to the Achilles tendon. Their results noted that, on average, the sural nerve and lesser saphenous veins were located 3.2 mm and 4.8 mm from the posterolateral portal, respectively. In terms of the posteromedial portal, they revealed that this was located on average 2.7 mm from the FHL tendon, 6.4 mm from the tibial nerve, 9.6 mm from the posterior tibial artery, and 17 mm from the medial calcaneal nerve.[11] These results were then corroborated by the later cadaveric study by Hendricks and colleagues.[12] They performed posterior arthroscopic ankle arthrodesis on 10 specimens using the same standard portals and found no incidence of neurovascular injury after assessing via open dissection.

Similarly, Balci and colleagues evaluated the structures at risk with posterior ankle arthroscopy, evaluating the effect of ankle joint position on the proximity of neurovascular structures. They used the same posteromedial and posterolateral portals as Sitler and colleagues and Hendricks and colleagues; however, they also placed the ankle joint in neutral, with 15° of dorsiflexion and 30° of plantarflexion. Findings suggested that in neutral, the posterolateral portal was 6 mm from the sural nerve and 1.6 mm from the peroneal tendons. The posteromedial portal was 2.11 mm from the FHL tendon and 6 mm from the posterior tibial artery. With dorsiflexion, the distance between the posteromedial portal and neurovascular bundle increased. This suggested that dorsiflexion of the ankle joint during portal placement may help protect the medial structures and help mitigate the overall risk of iatrogenic neurovascular injury.[13]

PATHOGENESIS

The term "impingement" in the orthopedic context refers to any abnormal entrapment or contact of structures resulting in pain or restricted motion.[14,15] As such, this pathology may be acute or chronic. Further, this anatomic region may involve multiple osseous and soft-tissue structures, either in isolation or in combination.[14]

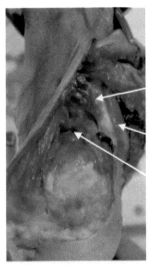

FHL Muscle Tendon

Tibial Nerve

Subtalar Joint

Fig. 1. Cadaveric dissection of the posterior arthroscopic landmarks and adjacent structures at risk. The FHL tendon and the posterior tibial neurovascular bundle are important anatomic structures medial to the posteromedial portal.

The most common cause of PAIS is often related to the posterolateral talar process and respective anatomic variants, including a Steida's process or symptomatic os trigonum. Again, this may be acute or chronic. Although a rare condition, os trigonum syndrome may occur acutely through hyperplantarflexion injury or chronic repetitive plantarflexion stress. As the talus rotates plantarly, the accessory ossicle or prominent posterolateral talar process becomes impinged between the inferior calcaneus and the tibial plafond. In a more acute context, abrupt hyperdorsiflexion of the foot about the ankle joint may produce traumatic avulsion of the posterolateral talar process (also termed a Shepherd fracture) or, in the case of an os trigonum, disruption of the synchondrosis connecting the accessory bone to the native talus.[2,5,14] In the more chronic setting, PAIS may result from previous fractures or degenerative arthritis that may lead to the formation of the ankle and subtalar osteophytes or loose bodies, capsular scarring, and reactive synovitis.[5,14]

In soft-tissue etiologies, the FHL tendon is commonly implicated; running between the medial and lateral posterior processes of the talus, it is commonly affected by tendinosis and tenosynovitis. Not only may the native soft tissue be impinged or hypertrophied by chronic repetitive plantarflexion injuries, but this may also lead to localized inflammation that gradually changes the adjacent FHL tendon.[2,14,16] Lastly, accessory musculature may also cause PAIS by either mechanical impingement or mass effect. Implicated accessory musculature includes peroneus quartus, flexor accessorius digitorum longus, peroneus calcaneus internus, tibiocalcaneus internus, accessory soleus, or a low-lying FHL muscle belly.[5] Although the above highlights some of the most common etiologies, an overview of the causes of PAIS reported in the literature is summarized in **Table 1**.

CLINICAL EVALUATION

Appropriate history and physical is performed to establish the nature, location, duration, onset, and aggravating and mitigating factors of the clinical complaint.[2] Generally, patients presenting with PAIS have a chief complaint of posterior lower ankle pain, worse during forced plantarflexion or propulsive push-off activities. There may be a clear pattern of provocative activities, including plantarflexion of the ankle joint or flexion and extension of the hallux. Physical examination may reveal reproducible pain produced with hyperplantarflexion, with or without posteromedial or posterolateral tenderness.[5,9]

Symptoms may be produced with resisted hallux plantarflexion, implicating FHL involvement. There may be a decrease in ankle joint range of motion, particularly in plantarflexion. If FHL involvement is apparent, there may be a reduction in hallux motion secondary to fibrosis and tendon adhesions. Diagnostic injections of local anesthetic with imaging guidance such as fluoroscopy or ultrasonography may help confirm diagnosis if pain relief is achieved with use. Differential diagnoses based on these findings can include fractures of the posterior tibiotalocalcaneal complex, osteochondral lesions of the talus and/or tibia, tarsal coalition, soft-tissue lesions, and tendon disorders inclusive of the peroneals and Achilles.[2]

A conventional three-view series of plain radiographs should be obtained, with the addition of a posterior impingement view. The posterior impingement view is a lateral, 25° external rotation, oblique view of the ankle, which has been demonstrated to show increased diagnostic accuracy in detecting an os trigonum as opposed to standard lateral views.[17,18] Plain films may identify the presence of posterolateral talar prominence or posterior impingement on the distal tibia (**Fig. 2**).

Advanced imaging, such as MRI and computed tomography (CT), may also be obtained. MRI may reveal inflammatory changes in the soft tissues of the posterior ankle, abnormal signal intensity in the lateral talar tubercle, os trigonum, bony prominence, effusion, synovitis, tenosynovitis, and/or concomitant chondral injury depending on the specific etiology. It may reveal FHL tenosynovitis, low-lying muscle belly, or aberrant accessory musculature (**Fig. 3**). In the absence of clear findings, the combined presence of bone marrow edema and posterior ankle synovitis may suggest the diagnosis of PAIS.[14,19] Sonography can be used to dynamically examine the gliding of the FHL tendon during passive dorsiflexion and plantarflexion of the ankle.[2] CT scan may reveal detailed morphology of bony lesions and more accurately establish the relation of bony structures. This may help identify if a fracture or nonunion is the primary cause of the impingement symptoms.

TREATMENT

As is the standard of care for most orthopedic processes, initial conservative management includes rest, ice, compressive therapy, elevation, anti-inflammatory

Table 1		
Posterior ankle impingement syndrome pathology		
Osseous Lesions	**Soft-Tissue Lesions**	**Aberrant Anatomy**
Stieda process os trigonum osteophytes Osteochondral lesion loose bodies chondromatosis		
	Flexor hallucis longus tenosynovitis synovitis Impingement of the joint capsule ligamentous hypertrophy	
		Peroneus quartus Flexor accessorius digitorum longus Peroneus calcaneus internus tibiocalcaneus internus accessory soleus
Subtalar coalition		Low-lying FHL muscle belly

medication, shoe gear modification, and avoidance of provocative activities. In some cases, a period of immobilization may be considered. Physical therapy may also be considered to address mobility, strength, and modification of sport-specific activity. Diagnostic and therapeutic injections of local anesthetic, corticosteroid, or combination may be administered, with careful avoidance of intratendinous corticosteroid injections. These injections may be performed with or without ultrasound guidance. Not only do these injections provide diagnostic utility, but also, if the patient responds positively to the injection, it may indicate a more favorable response to surgery. Although the above conservative treatment modalities may offer relief, oftentimes, the pain and symptoms are recalcitrant to these. It is suggested that approximately 40% of patients will eventually require surgical intervention due to intractable hindfoot pain.[17] Once the patient has completed and failed a 3- to 6-month course of conservative therapy, a surgical intervention must be considered.

Surgical intervention's goal in the PAIS setting involves resection of the causative anatomy.[14]

Surgical management of posterior ankle impingement was first described by Howse in 1982, detailing treatment of a posterior block of the ankle joint.[20] The traditional surgical intervention involved open posteromedial or posterolateral arthrotomy, which carries the risk of notable neurologic and vascular injuries, wound healing complications, and substantial recovery periods.[21] With the advancement of endoscopic technique, much of recent literature is devoted to arthroscopic and endoscopic approaches instead of open. In 2000, van Dijk and colleagues first detailed a two-portal technique of posterior ankle arthroendoscopy with patients in the prone position with favorable outcomes at 2-year follow-up. This method carefully and systematically avoided neurovascular injury.[9,10] Since then, posterior ankle impingement has become more routinely addressed with an endoscopic approach instead of an open

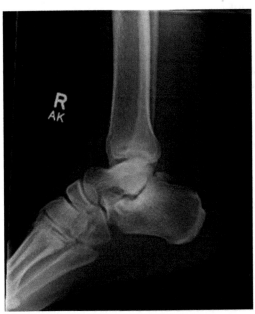

Fig. 2. Lateral radiograph of the ankle revealing fracture of the posterior process of the talus.

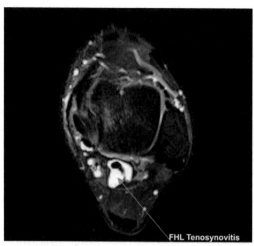

Fig. 3. Axial T2 MRI revealing increased signal intensity surrounding the FHL tendon, likely representing a pathologic tenosynovitis.

approach. The advantages of arthroscopy over open arthrotomy include decreased morbidity, less tissue disruption, less scarring, and the potential for a speedier recovery.[21] Once the decision to proceed with surgery has been made, a thorough preoperative medical work-up should be completed to clear the patient for elective surgery. It is essential to consider that the patient will be prone when reviewing pertinent medical history.

SURGICAL TECHNIQUE
Equipment

Standard arthroscopy equipment is used in posterior hindfoot arthroscopy. The surgeon may select either a 2.7 or 4.0 mm arthroscope with a 30° or 70° viewing angle, a 3.5 or 4.5 mm shaver for soft-tissue debridement, or a 4.0 mm aggressive shaver or burr for bony resection. All of the above may be selected based on surgeon preference. The authors of this article prefer a 4.0 mm 30° arthroscope. The authors also prefer to use saline set to 30 to 40 mm Hg for irrigation. However, some authors report fluid set to 50 to 60 mm Hg or even set to gravity.[2,17] A well-padded pneumatic thigh or high calf tourniquet may be used.

Positioning

The patient is transferred to the operating room table, positioned in a prone position. The operative limb is then elevated on several blankets, a pillow, or a ramp to raise the affected extremity above the contralateral. This allows for the increased working area and free movement for the arthroscopic equipment during the procedure and unrestricted movement and manipulation of the ankle joint. The pelvis should be bumped accordingly, allowing the foot to be positioned perpendicular to the floor, with the foot resting in a neutral position concerning the leg. The surface anatomy is then palpated and demarcated with an indelible marker. The first line is drawn, extending transversely from the fibula's tip to the ankle's medial aspect (Line 1). The medial and lateral borders of the Achilles tendon are then marked (Line 2), with the posteromedial and posterolateral portals drawn just above the intersection of the transverse line (Line

1) with the borders of the Achilles tendon. Lastly, a line is then drawn extending from the identified posterolateral portal site to the first interspace (Line 3), indicating the preferred direction of instrumentation (**Fig. 4**).

Arthroscopic Technique

The extremity is scrubbed, prepped, and draped in the usual aseptic manner. The posterolateral portal is established first, and the skin overlying the posterolateral portal is sharply incised with a blade, with care taken not to penetrate the subcutaneous layer. Dissection is then bluntly advanced to the level of bone with a mosquito hemostat, directed in the same orientation as the line drawn on the plantar aspect of the foot, toward the first interspace (Line 3). Once adequate dissection has been performed, a.

4.0 mm 30° arthroscope is introduced into the posterolateral portal and advanced to the level of bone. In the same plane as this posterolateral portal, the posteromedial portal is created just medial to the Achilles tendon, in an identical fashion to that described above. A hemostat is introduced through the posteromedial portal, and dissection is bluntly advanced until the hemostat is in contact with the arthroscope deep to the Achilles tendon. The arthroscope is maintained in its position directed toward the first interspace and is used as a guide for the hemostat to travel down to the level of bone, thereby avoiding injury to the neurovascular bundle. At this point, the posteromedial and posterolateral portals have now been established.

It is important to note that although posterior hindfoot arthroscopy is colloquially termed "arthroscopy", this is inaccurate. Instead, it truly is an endoscopic approach to an arthroscopic approach. At this point in the procedure, the equipment is extra-articular, and these extra-articular structures must be navigated to access the procedure's arthroscopic portion. The above hemostat is then replaced with a shaver. All working equipment is introduced through the posteromedial portal, directed laterally throughout the procedure. Some of the fat surrounding the arthroscope must be

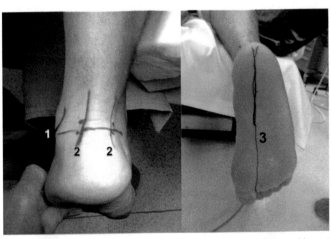

Fig. 4. Preoperative markings indicating appropriate surface anatomy and location for identified posteromedial and posterolateral portals. Line 1: A line drawn from the fibula's tip extending to the ankle joint's medial aspect in the transverse plane. Line 2: The medial and lateral borders of the Achilles tendon. Identified portals are indicated just above the intersection of lines 1 and 2. Line 3: Directed from the posterolateral portal toward the first webspace, indicating the appropriate direction of instrumentation.

excised to visualize the anatomic structures adequately. Once some of the periarticular fatty tissue is removed and adequate visualization has been obtained, anatomic landmarks can be identified. The most critical to identify is the.

FHL tendon (**Fig. 5**). The FHL tendon lies medial to the Stieda process along the posterior joint capsule. This is critical to visualize and work laterally to avoid compromise of the neurovascular structures, which lie medial to the tendon. Passive flexion and extension of the hallux can aid in this visualization. Ligamentous structures, including the posterior inferior tibiofibular ligament, posterior talofibular ligament, and calcaneofibular ligament, should be visualized laterally to the FHL. Deep into the capsule, the posterior subtalar and ankle joints can be visualized and inspected. The window visualized is defined laterally by the fibula and peroneal tendons, medially by the FHL tendon, neurovascular bundle, flexor digitorum longus tendon, posterior tibial tendon, and medial malleolus.

Many disorders can be addressed using this technique, in addition to PAIS. Posterior ankle and subtalar joint osteochondral lesions, subtalar and ankle arthritis, symptomatic loose osseous bodies, arthroscopic assisted fracture reduction, FHL or peroneal tenosynovitis, and excision of talocalcaneal coalitions may be addressed as well. The portals are then closed primarily, and the extremity is then sterilely dressed with dry dressings, with a cast, splint, or CAM boot applied if indicated.

Alternative Approaches

Although the above technique, initially described by van Dijk and colleagues in 2000, is the most widely used approach for posterior hindfoot endoscopy and arthroscopy, several other approaches have been detailed in the literature. In 2008, Horibe and colleagues described a different method for excision of a symptomatic os trigonum. They proposed using the posterolateral portal described by van Dijk and colleagues, but they used a posterolateral accessory portal instead of the van Dijk posteromedial portal.[10,22] This posterolateral accessory portal was placed just below the tip of the fibula, posterior to the peroneal tendons. Lui and colleagues, in 2016, reported an arthroscopic approach to decompression of posterior ankle impingement with the patient in the supine position. They reported using a posterolateral portal placed just posterior

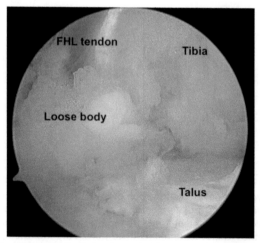

Fig. 5. Arthroscopic still image depicting loose body within the posterior ankle joint. Note the FHL tendon identified and the care taken to work laterally to the FHL tendon.

to the peroneal tendons at the ankle joint level in conjunction with a posteromedial portal placed just anterior to the posterior tibial tendon at the level of the ankle joint.[3] In 2022, Maffulli and colleagues described posterior extra-articular ankle endoscopy performed with the patient supine through double posteromedial portals. The posteromedial portals were placed just anterior to the anterior margin of the Achilles tendon, 45 to 50 mm apart, reporting favorable clinical and functional outcomes. The authors report no incidences of neurovascular compromise.[1] In addition to the above, reports have been published dictating the use of a posterolateral and anterolateral portal, double posterolateral portals, and a posterolateral and trans-Achilles portal.[23] Many of the above have fallen out of favor, and it is widely accepted that the above technique described by van Dijk and colleagues affords the most significant margin of safety from neurovascular structures.

Postoperative Protocols

As previously discussed, PAIS may be due to osseous structures, soft-tissue structures, or a combination thereof. Therefore, the postoperative protocol differs based on the type of procedure performed, and the pathology addressed. That said, most arthroscopic approaches involve an immediate range of motion of the ankle joint, prompt advances in weight-bearing status, with an expected return to training of approximately 5 weeks.[9,24] In the original literature described by van Dijk and colleagues in 2000, patients were placed in a soft dressing postoperatively following arthroscopic excision of symptomatic os trigonum.[10] Passive and active range of motion exercises of the ankle joint were initiated immediately following surgery, followed by weight-bearing as tolerated on postop day 3. Physical therapy was initiated 2 weeks postoperatively, and the patient returned to professional dancing after 6 weeks.[10]

Similarly, Gasparetto and colleagues[25] recommended weight-bearing tolerance for patients who underwent an FHL release, posterior impingement release, or osteochondral lesion debridement. Miyamoto and colleagues[26] allowed partial weight bearing with a soft dressing on a postoperative day 1. This trend of prompt range of motion and expeditious advances in weight-bearing follows the guidelines practiced by the authors of this article and is well supported in the literature on the surgical management of posterior impingement syndrome.[17] Physical therapy may or may not be indicated throughout the postoperative course. Literature has demonstrated an average return to total activity of 6 to 11 weeks postoperatively.[1,27,28]

DISCUSSION AND LITERATURE REVIEW

Initially described by van Dijk in 2000 as a case report, the two portal arthroendoscopic techniques described above yielded promising results, with a return to professional-level ballet activities at 6 weeks postoperatively.[10] Since 2000, van Dijk and colleagues have evaluated the above surgical approach. In 2006, they published a review of 146 endoscopic hindfoot procedures in 136 consecutive patients for whom the primary indication was PAIS. They reported a 1% complication rate, corresponding to a small area of transient hypoaesthesia in the heel pad. At the time, complication rates for open surgery in the setting of PAIS were reported to be 15% to 24% in the literature.[29]

Similarly, in 2008, Willits and colleagues[21] published a report on 15 patients with PAIS managed with posterior ankle arthroscopy. Five patients reported transient numbness or cutaneous irritation following surgery, which resolved by 4 months postoperatively. All but one patient was able to return to their previous level of sport at an average of 5.8 months.

The literature supports remarkably lower complication rates with endoscopic treatment as opposed to open treatment, and a much shorter return to activity accompanies the endoscopic approach. In 2012, Zengerink and colleagues established that the overall complication rate for hindfoot endoscopy was favorable and comparable to that of anterior ankle arthroscopy.[30] Zwiers and colleagues later assessed the endoscopic approach as compared with the open approach. Endoscopic approaches yielded lower complication rates, shorter recovery time, less postoperative pain, and comparable functional outcomes. Specifically, they reported an average of 11.3 weeks to return to sport, with a 1.8% significant complication rate in an endoscopic cohort.[27]

Similarly, Ribbans and colleagues[28] reported a 4.8% complication rate with arthroscopic approaches, as opposed to a 14.7% complication rate with open posterolateral approaches. This is corroborated by Georgiannos and colleagues,[31] who compared open versus endoscopic management for PAIS in their level 2 study. The endoscopic group returned to the previous sport level at an average of 7.12 weeks with a 3.8% complication rate, whereas the open group returned to the previous sport level at an average of 11.5 weeks with a 23% complication rate.

In 2017, van Dijk and colleagues[9] published a report on the current state of hindfoot arthroscopy. By this point, their approach had become the standard for posterior pathology, which is still true today. In this review, the authors reiterated that posterior ankle arthroscopy is considered safe and effective in treating PAIS. The most common complications reported include neurologic problems, sinus tract formation, and vascular damage. This is due to the proximity of the medial neurovascular bundle to the posteromedial portal and the posterolateral portal, which is close to the sural nerve. Reiterating the need for technical competency, Sugimoto and colleagues reported on the learning curve associated with posterior ankle arthroscopy as measured by surgical time. They reported an experience of 26 cases was required to demonstrate proficiency in posterior arthroscopies. Nevertheless, the midterm clinical outcomes, the patient-reported outcomes, and the return to sport remained consistent regardless of the order of the case in the series.[6]

It is well established in the literature that posterior ankle arthroendoscopy through the posterolateral and posteromedial portals described above is a safe and effective treatment of the management of the PAIS recalcitrant to conservative treatment modalities. Although risks include neurologic injury, this is principally sensory, frequently transient, and may be mitigated by an intimate knowledge of the local anatomy and surgeon experience.[16] Furthermore, this treatment offers a relatively expeditious return to sport in an active population.

CLINICS CARE POINTS

- When performing posterior ankle arthroscopy, care must be taken to stay within the anatomic window defined laterally by the fibula and peroneal tendons, and medially by the flexor hallucis longus tendon and neurovascular bundle.

- It is critical to review preoperative imaging carefully, assessing for anomalous anatomy.

- Posterior ankle arthroscopy is essentially an endoscopic approach to an arthroscopic technique. This procedure is initially instrument driven before direct visualization is able to be obtained.

- It is critical to respect the anatomic intimacy of the posterior ankle and subtalar joint capsules.

- When performing the procedure, all engine equipment should be introduced through the posteromedial portal, directed laterally to mitigate risk to the neurovascular structures.

DISCLOSURE

M.H. Theodoulou: Treace Medical, Avitus, Wishbone, Arthrex, Hemigard. M. Ravine has nothing to disclose.

REFERENCES

1. Maffulli N, Aicale R, Migliorini F, et al. The double posteromedial portals endoscopy for posterior ankle impingement syndrome in athletes. J Orthop Trauma 2022;23(28):1–6.
2. Theodoulou MH, Bohman L. Arthroscopic approach to posterior ankle impingement. Clin Podiatr Med Surg 2016;33:531–43.
3. Lui TH. Decompression of posterior ankle impingement with concomitant anterior ankle pathology by posterior ankle arthroscopy in the supine position. Arthrosc Tech 2016;5(5):e1191–6.
4. Pereira VF, Goncalves JP, Neves CMDSCC, et al. Posterior ankle impingement syndrome in athletes: surgical outcomes of a case series. Sco J Foot Ankle 2019;13(1):15–21.
5. Giannini S, Buda R, Mosca M, et al. Posterior ankle impingement. Foot Ankle Int 2013;34(3):459–65.
6. Sugimoto K, Isomoto S, Samoto N, et al. Arthroscopic treatment of posterior ankle impingement syndrome: mid-term clinical results and a learning curve. Sports Med Arthrosc Rehabil Ther Technol 2021;3(4):e1077–86.
7. Golano P, Vega J, Perez-Carro L, et al. Ankle anatomy for the arthroscopist. Part I: the portals. Foot Ankle Clin N Am 2006;11:253–73.
8. Golano P, Vega J, Perez-Carro L, et al. Ankle anatomy for the arthroscopist. Part II: role of the ankle ligaments in soft tissue impingement. Foot Ankle Clin N Am 2006;11:275–96.
9. Van Dijk CN, Vuurberg G, Batista J, et al. Posterior ankle arthroscopy: current state of the art. J ISAKOS 2017;2:269–77.
10. Van Dijk CN, Scholten PE, Krips R. A 2-portal endoscopic approach for diagnosis and treatment of posterior ankle pathology. Arthroscopy 2000;16(8):871–6.
11. Sitler DF, Amendola A, Bailey CS, et al. Posterior ankle arthroscopy: an anatomic study. J Bone Joint Surg Am 2002;84(5):763–9.
12. Hendrickx RPM, de Leeuw PAJ, Golano P, et al. Safety and efficiency of posterior arthroscopic ankle arthrodesis. Knee Surg Sports Traumatol Arthrosc 2015;23(8):2420–6.
13. Balci HI, Polat G, Dikmen G, et al. Safety of posterior ankle arthroscopy portals in different ankle positions: a cadaveric study. Knee Surg Sports Traumatol Arthrosc 2016;24(7):2119–23.
14. Lavery KP, McHale KJ, Rossy WH, et al. Ankle impingement. J Orthop Surg Res 2016;11(1):97.
15. Hayashi D, Roemer FW, D'Hooghe P, et al. Posterior ankle impingement in athletes: pathogenesis, imaging features and differential diagnoses. Eur J Radiol 2015;84(11):2231–41.

16. Chinnakkannu K, Femino JE, Glass N, et al. Posterior ankle and hindfoot arthroscopy: complications and posterior ankle impingement. Foot Ankle Orthop 2019; 4(4):1–2.
17. Yasui Y, Hannon CP, Hurley E, et al. Posterior ankle impingement syndrome: a systematic four-stage approach. World J Orthop 2016;7(10):657–63.
18. Wiegernick JI, Vroemen JC, van Dongen TH, et al. The posterior impingement view: an alternative conventional projection to detect bony posterior ankle impingement. Arthroscopy 2014;30(10):1311–6.
19. Cerezal L, Abascal F, Canga A, et al. MR Imaging of ankle impingement syndrome. AJR Am J Roentgenol 2003;181(2):551–9.
20. Howse AJG. Posterior block of the ankle joint in dancers. Foot Ankle Int 1982; 3(2):81–4.
21. Willits K, Sonneveld H, Amendola A, et al. Outcome of posterior ankle arthroscopy for hindfoot impingement. Arthroscopy 2008;24(2):196–202.
22. Horibe S, Kita K, Natsu-ume T, et al. A novel technique of arthroscopic excision of a symptomatic os trigonum. Arthroscopy 2008;24(1):121e1–4.
23. Smyth NA, Zwiers R, Wiegerinck JI, et al. Posterior hindfoot arthroscopy: a review. Am J Sports Med 2014;42(1):225–34.
24. Calder JD, Sexton SA, Pearce CJ. Returning to training and playing after posterior ankle arthroscopy for posterior impingement in elite professional soccer. Am J Sports Med 2010;38(1):120–4.
25. Gasparetto F, Collo G, Pisanu G, et al. Posterior ankle and subtalar arthroscopy: indications, technique, and results. Curr Rev Musculoskelet Med 2012;5(2): 164–70.
26. Miyamoto W, Takao M, Matsushita T. Hindfoot endoscopy for posterior ankle impingement syndrome and flexor hallucis longus tendon disorders. Foot Ankle Clin 2015;20(1):139–47.
27. Zwiers R, Wiegernick JI, Murawski CD, et al. Surgical treatment for posterior ankle impingement. Arthroscopy 2013;29(7):1263–70.
28. Ribbans WJ, Ribbans HA, Cruickshank JA, et al. The management of posterior ankle impingement syndrome in sport: a review. Foot Ankle Surg 2015; 21(1):1–10.
29. Van Dijk CN. Hindfoot endoscopy. Foot Ankle Clin N Am 2006;11:391–414.
30. Zengerink M, van Dijk CN. Complications in ankle arthroscopy. Knee Surg Sports Traumatol Arthrosc 2012;20:1420–31.
31. Georgiannos D, Bisbinas I. Endoscopic versus open excision of os trigonum for the treatment of posterior ankle impingement syndrome in an athletic population. Am J Sports Med 2017;45(6):1388–94.

Osteochondral Lesions of the Talus
The Questions We Would Like Answered

Sean T. Grambart, DPM[a,b,*], Alivia Passet, DPM[b],
Nathaniel Holte, DPM[b]

KEYWORDS

- Talar osteochondral lesion • Talus osteochondral lesion • Talar osteochondral defect
- Talus osteochondral defect • Microfracture

KEY POINTS

- The vascular anatomy of the talus is unique especially comparing the medial and lateral sides of the talus.
- Postoperative recovery should be patient specific but the trend is to maintain non–weight-bearing with range of motion.
- Overall healing process taking well over a year before it is complete.
- Return to sport can be expected within 4 to 6 months with a successful microfracture.

INTRODUCTION

Lesions to the articular cartilage are some of the most debilitating injuries due to the limited capacity for healing of the articular cartilage. The lack of blood supply, poor progenitor cell recruitment, and mitotic activity of hyaline cartilage makes osteochondral lesions challenging to manage.[1,2] Osteochondral lesions of the talus (OLTs) primarily develop from cartilage and subchondral bone changes, related to both ischemic and traumatic events.[3] Historically, the common mechanism of injury of the OLT normally occurs on the anterolateral side from ankle fracture or ankle sprain, whereas ischemic lesions occur on the posteromedial side.[4] OLTs have been reported to cause deep pain, stiffness, weakness, instability, and swelling of the ankle.[5] The unfortunate data suggest that conservative treatment with controlling the biologics, intra-articular injections, non–weight-bearing (NWB), and physiotherapy can resolve approximately 50% of symptomatic OLT.[6]

[a] Des Moines University College of Podiatric Medicine and Surgery, 3200 Grand Avenue, Des Moines, IA 50312, USA; [b] IMMC Foot and Ankle Surgery Residency Program, 3200 Grand Avenue, Des Moines, IA 50312, USA
* Corresponding author. Des Moines University Clinic, 3200 Grand Avenue, Des Moines, IA 50312.
E-mail address: Sean.Grambart@dmu.edu

Clin Podiatr Med Surg 40 (2023) 425–437
https://doi.org/10.1016/j.cpm.2023.02.004
0891-8422/23/© 2023 Elsevier Inc. All rights reserved.

podiatric.theclinics.com

Surgery is currently indicated with symptomatic OLTs that fail conservative treatment. The 2 primary treatment options consist of marrow stimulation with microfracture and retrograde drilling. Microfracturing is used to remove all unstable cartilage and subchondral bone to create stable vertical walls (**Fig. 1**). Penetration of the subchondral plate with the use of an osteochondral pick allows undifferentiated mesenchymal cells to form fibrocartilage around the lesion. The short-term effects of microfracturing have great results; however, the long-term effects of microfracturing worsen with time due to fibrocartilaginous deterioration.[7] There is also little evidence and agreement on whether repeat arthroscopy with microfracturing has a role in the management of failed previous procedures. Savva and colleagues[8] in a mini case series reported promising results with repeat arthroscopy for patients with recurrent symptoms of OLTs. Schafer and colleagues[9] determined similar results with 14 patients that had repeat microfractures for OLT and 12 of the 14 stated they would undergo the procedure again. However, Yoon and colleagues[10] determined that repeat microfracture had inferior outcomes compared with osteochondral autologous transplantation (OAT), with more than 60% of patients requiring further surgery.

Retrograde drilling is primarily used to treat subchondral cysts that have an intact overlying cartilage roof[11] (**Fig. 2**). There is currently conflicting information about retrograde drilling. A systematic review published in 2018 found that 68% to 100% of patients had a good outcome.[12] Jeong and colleagues published a case report of the 5-year follow-up of retrograde drilling for a subchondral cyst of OLT. They reported that the patient was admitted to the hospital due to severe ankle pain and the MRI showed arthritic changes to the ankle joint with multiple cystic formation in the talus. They concluded that there were 2 theories as to why their patient developed multiple subchondral cysts. The first theory is "Valve Mechanism" in which the subchondral cysts are caused by damage to the cartilage, which can function as a valve and allow intrusion of synovial joint fluid into the subchondral bone but not the opposite direction. The second theory is "Mucoid Degeneration" in which degeneration of connective tissue probably preceded by ischemia or aseptic necrosis. According to these 2 theories, the damaged articular cartilage needs to be debrided or subchondral cysts of the talus may reoccur.[13]

There is much debate on the consensus of OLTs in general. The authors' goal of this article is to ask and attempt to answer some common questions that relate to OLTs based on the entire perioperative period to aid the surgeon in improving patient outcomes.

How Does Ankle Instability Affect Osteochondral Lesions of the Talus?

Inversion injuries have long been implicated in the development of OLTs.[14,15] Lateral lesions seem to have an increased incidence due to trauma. Tol and colleagues[16]

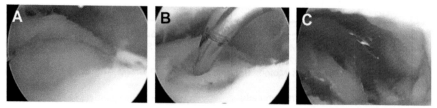

Fig. 1. OLT of the talus. (*A*) Lifting and fragmentation of the cartilage lesion. (*B*) Demonstration microfracture with the use of the osteochondral pick to perforate the subchondral plate. (*C*). Vascular reconstitution of the OLT after the microfracture.

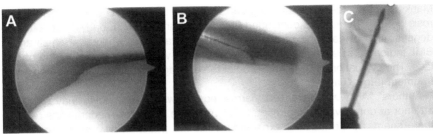

Fig. 2. (*A*) OLT with intact hyaline cartilage. (*B*) Probe showing the cartilage is intact but there is "softening" of the subchondral area. (*C*) Retrograde drilling of the lesion.

showed 93% of patients with lateral OLTs had a history of trauma compared with 62% of medial lesions. Surgeon intuition tells us that there should be a proportional increase in OLTs as ankle instability worsens. However, this may not be the case. Park and colleagues[17] in 2019 investigated the relationship between radiographic lateral ankle instability and OLTs following ankle inversion injuries. Their study included 195 patients with a history of inversion injuries of the ankle. Imaging for all patients included MRI and stress radiography. Radiographic lateral ankle instability was defined as tibiotalar tilt angle equal or greater than 10°. The presence of OLT was confirmed on MR images. Interestingly, the presence of radiographic lateral ankle instability (tibiotalar tilt angle equal or greater than 10°) showed an inverse relationship with that of OLT. An increased tibiotalar tilt angle was associated with lower incidence of OLT in the multiple regression analysis. The presence of OLT was actually associated with a decreased tibiotalar tilt angle using a binary logistic regression analysis.

Authors' "Answer": One could interpret the results of this study that the talus within the ankle mortise in a "stable" or constrained ankle joint lead to a more traumatic "impaction" of the talus within the mortise. We think this question opens the surgeon up for more questions. In a patient who undergoes an OLT repair with an ankle ligament repair, how "tight" should be the repaired ankle ligament. We think that this is an interesting area of potential research in the future.

How Accurate is MRI in the Prognosis of Healing?

MRI is often used as the primary advanced imaging modality when diagnosing and evaluating OLTs. It has the advantage of diagnosing any additional pathology that could influence surgical decision-making.[18] MRI may also have the added advantage of evaluating the healing potential of the OLT preoperatively. Bone marrow edema is commonly observed in the subchondral bone on MRI. Nakasa and colleagues[19] in 2018 investigated the relationship between bone marrow edema and cartilage degeneration in OLT. Thirty-three ankles with OLTs all underwent computed tomography (CT) and MRI and had operative treatment. The ankles were divided into 2 groups, with or without sclerosis. The sclerosis was evaluated in the host bone just below the osteochondral fragment (nonsclerosis group and sclerosis group). The area of the bone marrow edema was compared between the 2 groups. Biopsies of the osteochondral fragment from 20 ankles were performed during surgery, and the correlation between the bone marrow edema and cartilage degeneration was analyzed. The other 13 ankles had the CT and MRI compared with the arthroscopic findings. The nonsclerosis group area of bone marrow edema was significantly larger than that in the sclerosis group. In the histologic analysis, there was a significant and moderate correlation between the Mankin score and the area of bone marrow lesion (BML). The mean

Mankin score in the nonsclerosis group was significantly lower than that in the sclerosis group. The authors concluded that a large area of BML on MRI exhibited low degeneration of cartilage of the osteochondral fragment, whereas a small area of BML indicated sclerosis of the subchondral bone with severe degeneration of cartilage. The evaluation of BML may predict the cartilage condition of the osteochondral fragment (**Figs. 3** and **4**).

Authors' "Answer": Increased marrow edema with MRI imaging may warrant an attempt at conservative treatment. However, once the marrow edema has resolved, there seems to be minimal expectations on the patient's own ability to heal the OLT. The MRI with obvious osteochondral deficit or cystic changes with an increased signal intensity do not indicate healing.

Does the Size of the Osteochondral Lesion of the Talus Matter?

This is one of the most heavily debated topics in treating OLTs. Many surgeons think that because microfracture or retrograde drilling is less invasive, this should be attempted on all OLTs as a first-line treatment. However, larger lesions have worse outcomes, which would be expected (**Fig. 5**). This was emphasized in 2009, when Choi and colleagues[20] evaluated the prognostic significance and optimal measures of defect size in OLT as treated with arthroscopy. One hundred twenty ankles underwent arthroscopic marrow stimulation treatment of OLT and were evaluated for prognostic factors. Clinical failure was defined as patients' having osteochondral transplantation or an AOFAS Ankle-Hindfoot Scale score less than 80. Of the 120 ankles, 8 ankles (6.7%) required osteochondral transplantation, and 22 ankles (18.4%) were considered failures because of AOFAS scores less than 80. They concluded that the initial defect size is an important and easily obtainable prognostic factor in OLTs and so may serve as a basis for preoperative surgical decisions. A cutoff point exists regarding the risk of clinical failure at a defect area of approximately 150 mm^2 as calculated from MRI.

A recent systematic review has challenged the traditionally quoted 150 mm^2 for failure of marrow stimulation techniques.[21] Twenty-five studies with 1868 ankles were included. The mean area was 103.8 $\pm$ 10.2 mm^2 in 20 studies, and the mean diameter

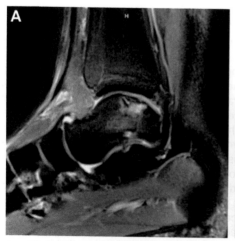
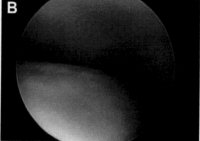

Fig. 3. (*A*) MRI showing a large area of increased signal intensity under the OLT, which indicates minimal sclerosis and good vascular supply for potential healing of the OLT. (*B*) Arthroscopic view of the lesion showing intact hyaline cartilage.

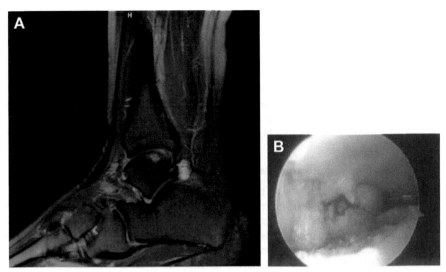

Fig. 4. (*A*) MRI showing a small area of increased signal intensity indicating sclerosis of the lesion and minimal chance to heal. (*B*) Arthroscopic view of the OLT with degeneration of the hyaline cartilage.

was 10.0 ± 3.2 mm in 5 studies. The mean American Orthopedic Foot and Ankle Society score improved from 62.4 ± 7.9 preoperatively to 83.9 ± 9.2 at a mean 54.1-month follow-up in 14 studies reporting both preoperative and postoperative scores. The study had a mean follow-up of more than 2 years. A significant correlation was found in 3 studies, with a mean lesion area of 107.4 ± 10.4 mm^2. The authors'

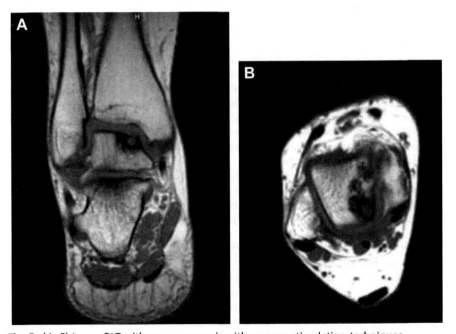

Fig. 5. (*A, B*) Large OLT with poor prognosis with marrow stimulation techniques.

assessment of the currently available data does suggest that bone marrow stimulation (BMS) may best be reserved for OLT sizes less than 107.4 mm^2 in area and/or 10.2 mm in diameter.

Authors' "Answer": It seems that the often quoted 150 mm(2) may be overestimated on the size in which marrow stimulation may fail. The authors recommend marrow stimulation as a first line in OLTs in which the mean area is less than 110 mm^2. Although, we discuss the advantages and disadvantages of marrow stimulation in larger lesions, with the patients as many still will elect to try a less-invasive procedure as the first line of treatment even knowing that there is an increased risk of further surgery.

Does the Surrounding Anatomy Matter?

The authors think that this could be one of the more interesting takes on healing of OLTs. Surgeons treat lateral and medial talar lesions very similarly with surgical technique and instrumentation but could the anatomy and thus the healing biology be different between these areas. This seems to be an area that could alter the surgeons' approach to OLTs. Wang and colleagues[22] explored the optimal drilling depth and direction for OLTs based on a 3-dimensional vascular microarchitecture model constructed. They perfused 12 talus specimens using a contrast agent and then scanned the specimens with a micro-CT. The talar dome was divided into 9 zones, and the vessel densities were measured at the subchondral depths of 0 to 5 mm, 5 to 10 mm, and 10 to 15 mm in each zone. They found that the vessel density of the 0 to 5-mm depth was lower than that of the 5 to 10-mm and 10 to 15-mm depths but no significant difference was found between the 5 to 10-mm and 10 to 15-mm depths. The vessel density in the 5 to 10-mm depth of medial talar dome was similar to that of the adjacent zones. Vessel density in the 5 to 10-mm depth around the lateral talar dome was higher in the anterior and medial side. With a retrograde approach, the anterolateral approach disturbed the main intraosseous vessels from the tarsal canal-tarsal sinus, causing extensive vascular compromise in the talus neck and body, whereas the posterolateral approach disturbed only the vessels near the tunnel. The authors concluded that the vessel density changed greatly from the subchondral 0 to 5-mm to the 5 to 10-mm depth. The vessel densities of the 5 to 10-mm depth around the medial talar dome were similar, whereas the anterior and medial side of the lateral talar dome was better vascularized. The posterolateral approach caused less vascular damage than the anterolateral approach. From a surgeon's standpoint, especially with a microfracture approach, the depth that the subchondral plate is perforated may not be the ideal depth to optimize vascular influx with the current arthroscopic instruments that are commonly used as the preferable depth is 5 to 10-mm below the subchondral plate.

Authors' "Answer": This is an interesting topic. Most of the osteochondral picks that are used in surgery do not penetrate the 5 to 10-mm ideal vascular supply. In view of this study, we do use different instrumentation with microfracture to make sure we access the vascular area (**Figs. 6** and **7**).

Do Adjuvants Augment the Healing Process?

Biologic augmentation

There are numerous studies that discuss the use of biologics to aid in the regeneration of hyaline-like articular cartilage, a tissue known to have limited regenerative capacity.[23] Platelet rich plasma (PRP) is one biologic that has gained momentum. PRP is composed of the patient's own platelets and growth factors that can help stimulate cartilage regrowth and extracellular matrix synthesis. PRP can act as an adjunct to

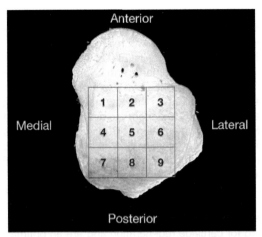

Fig. 6. Superior articular surface of the talus divided into 9 zones. (*Adapted from* Wang D, et al. Vascular Compromising Effect of Drilling for Osteochondral Lesions of the Talus: A Three-Dimensional Micro-Computed Tomography Study. Arthroscopy. 2019 Oct;35(10):2930-2937.)

cartilage repair by decreasing inflammatory mediators, increasing collagen synthesis and recruiting mesenchymal stem cells (MSCs).[24] A systematic review of the clinical trials of PRP demonstrated that PRP promotes the recovery of function and reduces pain in OLT when used as an adjunctive procedure to microfracturing or conservative treatment.[25]

Hyaluronic acid (HA) is a glycosaminoglycan that is located within synovial fluid. In water, HA forms a viscous gel-like substance that has nociceptive blocking properties. In vitro studies have proven that HA has promoted cartilage regeneration and chondrocyte proliferation.[24] A systematic review of randomized controlled trials done in 2022 evaluated 3 randomized studies with a total of 132 patients and determined

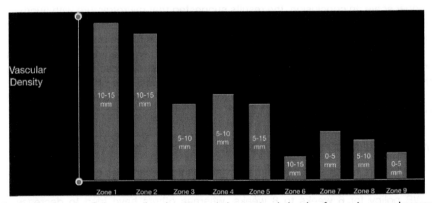

Fig. 7. Bar graph of the vascular density and the optimal depth of vascular vessels corresponding to the zones of the talus from **Fig. 6**. Zone 1 and Zone 2 have the greatest vascular density with the ideal depth of 10 to 15 mm. Zone 6 has the least vascular density with the ideal depth of 10 to 15 mm. (*Interpretation from* Wang D, et al. Vascular Compromising Effect of Drilling for Osteochondral Lesions of the Talus: A Three-Dimensional Micro-Computed Tomography Study. Arthroscopy. 2019 Oct;35(10):2930-2937.)

that HA injections as an adjunctive to microfracturing for OLT proved that in the short-term follow-up, there was a statistical significance and greater improvement in VAS-pain and functional scores compared with microfracture alone.[26]

Embryonic-derived mesenchymal cells (EMCs) are pluripotent stem cells that have the ability to differentiate into any primary germ layer. Pluripotency is an unlimited self-renewal, and this is what distinguishes EMC from other stem cells. The application of EMC for cartilage repair is still in its infancy stages. Currently, there are very few studies in vitro that use the EMC and there are no known studies in the foot and ankle that have used EMC as an augmentation.[24] Cheng and colleagues[27] used EMCs that were encapsulated in a fibrin gel for an osteochondral lesion of the patellar groove. The authors observed upregulation of chondrogenic genes. The use of EMCs raises ethical concerns because they are derived from embryos.

Bone marrow aspirate (BMA) concentrations contain adult MSCs and other tissues. These stem cells are multipotent and have the ability to only differentiate along connective tissue lineages: chondrocytes, osteoblasts, and myocytes. BMA stem cells are commonly used for cartilage regeneration and are an optimal option due to their accessibility.[24] Fortier and colleagues[28] have demonstrated that the use of BMA in preclinical trials in equine models with microfracturing can be used for full-thickness cartilage defects. The histological and MRI analysis showed superior healing from the BMA and microfracture compared with microfracture alone.

Biologic use is an up-and-coming augmentation supplementation to current procedures. Wen and colleagues[29] published a systematic review and meta-analysis on the 492 patients from 1950 to 2020. The 10 studies were only randomized controlled trials, quasi-randomized controlled trials, and observational studies (retrospective and prospective) that compared microfracturing along versus microfracturing plus biologic augmentation. The augmentation was defined as addition of MSCs, bone marrow aspirate concentration, PRP, hyaluronic acid, or autologous matrix-induced chondrogenesis after microfracture technique for OLTs. Their outcome was that microfracture plus augmentation was superior to microfracture alone in final AOFAS score, AOFAS change scores, visual analog scale (VAS) change scores, and magnetic resonance observation of cartilage repair tissue score, decreased complications and decreased in revisions. There were no significant differences in final VAS score and Tegner scale. In conclusion, the results suggested that microfracture with augmentation were superior for OLTs. To our knowledge, there are no head-to-head randomized control trials that directly compare the use of biologics to one another.

Authors' "Answer": This is an interesting topic. We have used different adjuvants to try and aid in the healing process. There are minimal randomized studies on this topic that need to be explored to get a definitive answer. Cost also plays a role in this decision to add adjuvants to try and promote healing. Further information is needed on this topic.

WHAT IS THE BEST POSTOP PROTOCOL?

Microfracture treatment or bone marrow stimulation techniques currently do not have a gold standard for the postoperative protocol. Most surgeons will adhere to a strict NWB policy for 6 weeks to 8 weeks, whereas others have tried to decrease the NWB period to help increase patient satisfaction, quality of life, and decrease the potential loss of work.[30]

Danilkowicz and colleagues[31] published a retrospective review of 69 patients looking at 2 groups of patients. Early weight-bearing (EWB) had 18 patients and delayed weight-bearing (DWB) had 51 patients. There were no statistical differences between their age, race, weight, height, smoking status, or lesion size. The outcome of the study was that the EWB group had improved VAS pain scores from 4.40 to 0.67 compared with the NWB group with a VAS pain score from 6.33 to 2.55 at final follow-up, this was of significance. The surgical management of OLTs is a challenging process for both surgeon and patient. The conclusion was no difference in VAS, ROM, or complications when allowing EWB in a CAM boot at 2 weeks versus NWB for 6 weeks. These results were similar to Deal and colleagues[32] in 2019 that published a prospective randomized trial of EWB versus DWB for microfractures of OLTs. In this trial, 18 subjects were in the EWB and 20 in the DWB. At the first surgical postoperative visit, the EWB group was placed in a CAM boot and had unrestricted WB at that time, whereas the DWB group was instructed to remain NWB for an additional 4 weeks. At a 6-week follow-up, the EWB patients demonstrated significant improvement in AAOS foot and Ankle Questionnaire scores compared with the DWB group. The preceding follow-ups through the 2 years did not show statistical significance between the AAOS scores or pain scores. In their conclusion, EWB with microfracture for OLTs was associated with improved AAOS scores in the short term but there was no statistical significance in the long term. Song and colleagues[33] published a meta-analysis and systematic review in 2021 comparing the results of EWB versus DWB after microfracture for OLT. This study compared 5 previously published articles with a total of 283 patients that were evaluated at 3 months, 6 months, 12 months, and 24 months postoperatively for VAS score and AOFAS scale score. There was no statistical significance between EWB and DWB for VAS score and AOFAS scale score at the 3-month, 6-month, 12-month, and 24-month follow-ups.

Authors' "Answer": There is still no set standard for postoperative protocol for microfracturing for OLTs. There seems to be a trend in improvement in patients at the 4-week follow-up for EWB compared with DWB but this could have been due to patients having improved quality of life with being able to WB in a CAM boot versus staying strictly NWB. We typically recommend protected weight-bearing for smaller size lesions at 2 weeks and larger lesion at 4 to 6 weeks. Much of this discussion is still anecdotal and more research is needed.

WHAT IS THE EXPECTED RETURN TO SPORT/ACTIVITIES AND WHEN?

Treatment options for athletes usually consist of surgical intervention from microfracturing for first line small and medium OLT to OATS or allografts larger lesions.[21] One of the main questions that many athletes will ask is when they can return to sports activity after surgical treatment. The current evidence for surgical intervention of OLT is very scarce for microfracturing on elite athletes. Lee and colleagues[34] in 2021 published a case series on lesion size being able to predict when young elite athletes can return to play after microfracturing for OLT. They evaluated 41 patients with a mean follow-up of 54.9 months. A total of 41 patients, 20 played professional league, 11 were collegiate athletes, and 10 were high-school students preparing for professional sports as their primary career. The clinical outcome for all the patients was significantly improved at final follow-up for FAOS, AOFAS, and VAS scores. All 41 (100%) patients were initially able to return to sports activity. However, 74.4% were able to continue their sports careers for at least 2 years. Eight out of 10 (80.0%) high school students, 8 out of 11 (72.7%) were university athletes, and 13 out of 20 (65.0%) were professional athletes who were able to return to play. The only significant factor that affected return to play was lesion size 84.0 mm². All athletes returned to competition at an average of 5.45 months and 74.4% were able to return to play. D'Ambrosi and colleagues[35] also came to the same conclusion in their study where all patients underwent arthroscopic autologous matrix-induced chondrogenesis and they determined that 80.8% of patients returned to preinjury sport with an average follow-up of 42.6 months.

Hurley and colleagues[36] systematically reviewed the literature to evaluate the reported rehabilitation protocols, return to play guidelines, and subsequent rates and timing of return to play following bone marrow stimulation for OLTs. Fifty-seven studies with 3072 ankles were included, with a mean age of 36.9 years, and a mean follow-up of 46.0 months. The mean rate of return to play was 86.8%, and the mean time to return to play was 4.5 months. Rehabilitation protocols varied greatly between the studies. Range of motion exercises were allowed to begin in the first week (46.2%), and second week postoperatively (23.1%). The most reported time to start partial weight-bearing was the first week (38.8%), and the most frequently reported time of commencing full weight-bearing was 6 weeks (28.8%). Surgeons most often allowed return to play at 4 months (37.5%).

Authors' "Answer": Expectations for athletes must be reasonable, and return to sport is normally done under the guidance of trainers or physical therapist. We recommend discussing a 4 to 6-month return on primary lesions.

What Is the Overall Prognosis?

Patients want to know when they will be back to "normal" or see the most improvement. Kim and colleagues followed 64 patients that underwent microfracture in patients with OLT. Follow-up for more than 3 years. They analyzed and compared the clinical outcome changes according to time, the visual analog scale (VAS), and AOFAS ankle-hindfoot scores were evaluated every 3 months up to 1 year postoperatively and every 1 year after. The analysis contained outcome differences based on the lesion size, lesion location, lesion containment, presence of cyst and bone marrow edema, age, sex, and obesity. Both the VAS and AOFAS preoperative and final follow-up VAS scores significantly improved. The overall success rate for arthroscopic microfracture in this study was 88.6%. The average postoperative VAS scores at 3, 6, 9, 12, 24, and 36 months were 3.7, 2.5, 2.0, 1.6, 1.2, and 1.3. The average AOFAS scores during the same time increments were 74.7, 80.5, 84.3, 88.3, 91.1, and 90.8. No clinical outcome differences based on the lesion size, lesion containment, presence of cyst and bone marrow edema, age, sex, and obesity were observed. The authors concluded that symptomatic improvement early after arthroscopic microfracture for OLT was observed continuously for up to 2 years postoperatively. Symptom improvement was maintained without worsening for up to 3 years after surgery.

After 3 years, a microfracture repair seems to maintain its healing with midsize lesions. Choi and colleagues[37] showed good intermediate-term functional outcomes with microfracture for OLTs. One hundred sixty-seven ankles that underwent arthroscopic microfracture for small-to-midsized OLT with a mean lesion size of 73 mm^2. AOFAS ankle-hindfoot scale showed an improvement from 71.0 points preoperatively to 89.5 points at the final follow-up. The VAS score showed an improvement from 6.2 points preoperatively to 1.7 points at the final follow-up. The mean SF-36 score improved from 62.4 points preoperatively to 76.2 points at the final follow-up. Twenty-two ankles (13.3%) underwent repeat arthroscopic surgery for the evaluation of repaired cartilage status.

Authors' "Answer": OLTs take time to heal. We anticipate that most surgeons have a tendency to consider a marrow stimulation failure at a time shorter than 2 years postoperative. If patients continue to improve, time must be given to allow the area to heal. However, if the patient worsens especially in the first 6 months, then the repair will not likely improve.

CLINICS CARE POINTS

- MRI is a vital tool used to assess the healing of OLTs. Decreased marrow edema is an indicator of decreased ability to heal compared with an increased signal intensity indicating a higher propensity to heal.
- Worsening symptoms within 6 months of the procedure is an indicator of an unsuccessful microfracture.
- Smaller lesions with microfracture can typically begin protected weight-bearing at 2 weeks, whereas larger lesions need 4 to 6 weeks on non–weight-bearing before protected weight-bearing can be initiated.

DISCLOSURE

The authors have nothing to disclose.

REFERENCES

1. Dowthwaite GP, Bishop JC, Redman SN, et al. The surface of articular cartilage contains a progenitor cell population. J Cell Sci 2004;117(Pt 6):889–97.
2. Alford JW, Cole BJ. Cartilage restoration, part 2: techniques, outcomes, and future directions. Am J Sports Med 2005;33(3):443–60.
3. Badekas T, Takvorian M, Souras N. Treatment principles for osteochondral lesions in foot and ankle. Int Orthop 2013;37(9):1697–706.
4. Navid DO, Myerson MS. Approach alternatives for treatment of osteochondral lesions of the talus. Foot Ankle Clin 2002;7(3):635–49.
5. Hintermann B, Boss A, Schafer D. Arthroscopic findings in patients with chronic ankle instability. Am J Sports Med 2002;30(3):402–9.
6. Shearer C, Loomer R, Clement D. Nonoperatively managed stage 5 osteochondral talar lesions. Foot Ankle Int 2002;23(7):651–4.
7. Toale J, Shimozono Y, Mulvin C, et al. Midterm outcomes of bone marrow stimulation for primary osteochondral lesions of the talus: a systematic review. Orthop J Sports Med 2019;7(10). 2325967119879127.
8. Savva N, Jabur M, Davies M, et al. Osteochondral lesions of the talus: results of repeat arthroscopic debridement. Foot Ankle Int 2007;28(6):669–73.
9. Schafer KA, Cusworth BM, Kazarian GS, et al. Outcomes following repeat ankle arthroscopy and microfracture for osteochondral lesions of the talus. Foot Ankle Spec 2022. https://doi.org/10.1177/19386400221079203.
10. Yoon HS, Park YJ, Lee M, et al. Osteochondral autologous transplantation is superior to repeat arthroscopy for the treatment of osteochondral lesions of the talus after failed primary arthroscopic treatment. Am J Sports Med 2014;42(8):1896–903.
11. Shimozono Y, Brown AJ, Batista JP, et al. Subchondral pathology: proceedings of the international consensus meeting on cartilage repair of the ankle. Foot Ankle Int 2018;39(1_suppl):48S–53S.
12. Dahmen J, Lambers KTA, Reilingh ML, et al. No superior treatment for primary osteochondral defects of the talus. Knee Surg Sports Traumatol Arthrosc 2018;26(7):2142–57.
13. Jeong SY, Kim JK, Lee KB. Is retrograde drilling really useful for osteochondral lesion of talus with subchondral cyst?: a case report. Medicine (Baltim) 2016;95(49):e5418.

14. Murawski CD, Kennedy JG. Operative treatment of osteochondral lesions of the talus. J Bone Joint Surg Am 2013;95(11):1045–54.
15. Stufkens SA, Knupp M, Horisberger M, et al. Cartilage lesions and the development of osteoarthritis after internal fixation of ankle fractures: a prospective study. J Bone Joint Surg Am 2010;92(2):279–86.
16. Tol JL, Struijs PA, Bossuyt PM, et al. Treatment strategies in osteochondral defects of the talar dome: a systematic review. Foot Ankle Int 2000;21(2):119–26.
17. Park BS, Chung CY, Park MS, et al. Inverse relationship between radiographic lateral ankle instability and osteochondral lesions of the talus in patients with ankle inversion injuries. Foot Ankle Int 2019;40(12):1368–74.
18. Verhagen RA, Maas M, Dijkgraaf MG, et al. Prospective study on diagnostic strategies in osteochondral lesions of the talus. Is MRI superior to helical CT? J Bone Joint Surg Br 2005;87(1):41–6.
19. Nakasa T, Ikuta Y, Sawa M, et al. Relationship between bone marrow lesions on mri and cartilage degeneration in osteochondral lesions of the talar dome. Foot Ankle Int 2018;39(8):908–15.
20. Choi WJ, Park KK, Kim BS, et al. Osteochondral lesion of the talus: is there a critical defect size for poor outcome? Am J Sports Med 2009;37(10):1974–80.
21. Ramponi L, Yasui Y, Murawski CD, et al. Lesion size is a predictor of clinical outcomes after bone marrow stimulation for osteochondral lesions of the talus: a systematic review. Am J Sports Med 2017;45(7):1698–705.
22. Wang D, Shen Z, Fang X, et al. Vascular compromising effect of drilling for osteochondral lesions of the talus: a three-dimensional micro-computed tomography study. Arthroscopy 2019;35(10):2930–7.
23. Becher C, Driessen A, Hess T, et al. Microfracture for chondral defects of the talus: maintenance of early results at midterm follow-up. Knee Surg Sports Traumatol Arthrosc 2010;18(5):656–63.
24. Hogan MV, Hicks JJ, Chambers MC, et al. Biologic adjuvants for the management of osteochondral lesions of the talus. J Am Acad Orthop Surg 2019;27(3): e105–11.
25. Yausep OE, Madhi I, Trigkilidas D. Platelet rich plasma for treatment of osteochondral lesions of the talus: a systematic review of clinical trials. J Orthop 2020;18:218–25.
26. Dilley JE, Everhart JS, Klitzman RG. Hyaluronic acid as an adjunct to microfracture in the treatment of osteochondral lesions of the talus: a systematic review of randomized controlled trials. BMC Musculoskelet Disord 2022;23(1):313.
27. Cheng A, Kapacee Z, Peng J, et al. Cartilage repair using human embryonic stem cell-derived chondroprogenitors. Stem Cells Transl Med 2014;3(11): 1287–94.
28. Fortier LA, Potter HG, Rickey EJ, et al. Concentrated bone marrow aspirate improves full-thickness cartilage repair compared with microfracture in the equine model. J Bone Joint Surg Am 2010;92(10):1927–37.
29. Wen HJ, Zhu SY, Tan HB, et al. Augmented microfracture technique versus microfracture in talar cartilage restoration: a systematic review and meta-analysis. J Foot Ankle Surg 2021;60(6):1270–9.
30. Hurst JM, Steadman JR, O'Brien L, et al. Rehabilitation following microfracture for chondral injury in the knee. Clin Sports Med 2010;29(2):257–65, viii.
31. Danilkowicz RM, Grimm NL, Zhang GX, et al. Impact of early weightbearing after ankle arthroscopy and bone marrow stimulation for osteochondral lesions of the talus. Orthop J Sports Med 2021;9(9). 23259671211029883.

32. Deal JB Jr, Patzkowski JC, Groth AT, et al. Early vs delayed weightbearing after microfracture of osteochondral lesions of the talus: a prospective randomized trial. Foot Ankle Orthop 2019;4(2). 2473011419838832.
33. Song M, Li S, Yang S, et al. Is Early or delayed weightbearing the better choice after microfracture for osteochondral lesions of the talus? A meta-analysis and systematic review. J Foot Ankle Surg 2021;60(6):1232–40.
34. Lee KT, Song SY, Hyuk J, et al. Lesion size may predict return to play in young elite athletes undergoing microfracture for osteochondral lesions of the talus. Arthroscopy 2021;37(5):1612–9.
35. D'Ambrosi R, Villafane JH, Indino C, et al. Return to sport after arthroscopic autologous matrix-induced chondrogenesis for patients with osteochondral lesion of the talus. Clin J Sport Med 2019;29(6):470–5.
36. Hurley ET, Shimozono Y, McGoldrick NP, et al. High reported rate of return to play following bone marrow stimulation for osteochondral lesions of the talus. Knee Surg Sports Traumatol Arthrosc 2019;27(9):2721–30.
37. Choi SW, Lee GW, Lee KB. Arthroscopic microfracture for osteochondral lesions of the talus: functional outcomes at a mean of 6.7 years in 165 consecutive ankles. Am J Sports Med 2020;48(1):153–8.

Subtalar Joint Arthroscopy

Jonathon Srour, DPM, AACFAS[a], Laurence Rubin, DPM[b],*

KEYWORDS

- Subtalar joint • Arthroscopy • Fluoroscopy • Arthroscopic Fracture Reduction
- Foot and Ankle • STJ Arthroscopy

KEY POINTS

- Subtalar arthroscopy is useful for a variety of pathologies and adjunctive treatments.
- The anatomy and approach is more challenging than ankle arthroscopy but, with proper training, can be equally as useful.
- The foot and ankle surgeon should be mindful of the complex anatomy and potential complications of subtalar arthroscopy.
- With continued research and training, the foot and ankle surgeon can improve patient outcomes with the use of subtalar arthroscopy.

Subtalar joint arthroscopy, which was first described in 1985 by Parisien and colleagues is related to ankle joint arthroscopy in the proximity of the portals but technical aspects can be significantly more challenging given the unique anatomy. There are four articular surfaces: the anterior facet, middle facet, posterior facet, and the articular surface of the talonavicular joint anteriorly. The addition of intra-articular and periarticular ligaments as well as the roots of the extensor retinaculum provide an even greater challenge to the arthroscopist.[1]

The joint can be accessed via both anterior and posterior approaches. The anterior approach is used more commonly given both the preponderance of pathologies for which it can treat as well as the fact that it presents less challenging anatomy. The posterior portal, while useful for certain conditions, is complicated by a narrow joint space and a deceptive proximity to the ankle joint. Similar to the ankle joint, there are both diagnostic and therapeutic indications for subtalar joint arthroscopy and these have recently increased. This article will focus on both techniques as well as various indications for surgery.[1]

DIAGNOSTIC TESTS

As with any surgical procedure, the correct diagnosis is vital to a successful subtalar joint arthroscopy. Through comparative palpation, neighboring anatomical structures can be ruled out as contributory to the patient's hindfoot pain. These include the

[a] Tier 1 Orthopedic and Neurosurgical Institute, 105 S. Willow Avenue, Cookeville, TN 38501, USA; [b] Foot and Ankle Specialists of Virginia, 7016 Lee Park Road, Ste 105, Mechanicsville, VA 23111, USA
* Corresponding author.
E-mail address: lgrubin1413@gmail.com

Clin Podiatr Med Surg 40 (2023) 439–444
https://doi.org/10.1016/j.cpm.2023.03.001
0891-8422/23/© 2023 Elsevier Inc. All rights reserved.

peroneal tendons, calcaneal–cuboid joint, anterior talofibular ligament and calcaneal fibular ligament, sural nerve, and the lateral gutter of the ankle joint. Although they should generally be obtained before a subtalar joint arthroscopy, plain film radiographs are generally only going to show subtalar joint pathology later in the degenerative process when an arthroscopic debridement may no longer be warranted. A selective block of the subtalar joint is extremely helpful in confirming the diagnosis. The needle is introduced to the joint at the sinus tarsi and the local anesthetic is infiltrated. The patient resumes their daily activities and is instructed to pay attention to which activities they can once again perform without pain. If the pathology is intraarticular, the patient should achieve short-term relief of their pain. Short-acting and long-acting steroids like dexamethasone and triamcinolone can also be combined with the injection for a longer-term therapeutic benefit.

Advanced imaging like computed tomography (CT) and MRI may be helpful but must be used in conjunction with the physical exam. Taking into account that MRI is a preferred way to evaluate non-ossified structures, such as articular cartilage, marrow tissue, and synovial fluid, Zaedi and colleagues developed a scoring system for arthritic changes to the joint to be used for assessment and monitoring of patients with suspected and known degenerative disease.[17] Additionally, increases in the T2 and associated decreases in the T1 signal can suggest contusions of the bone marrow, microtrabecular fractures, and reactive trabecular changes from altered biomechanics.[2] Similarly, Powell and Cooper suggested that MRI could indicate the location and size of chondral lesions which could guide surgical management with arthroscopy of the subtalar joint.[3]

CONSERVATIVE TREATMENT

Subtalar joint symptoms have generally been present for a significant period upon presentation to the foot and ankle surgeon. For more acute injuries: ice, elevation, and immobilization are recommended. non-steroidal anti-inflammatory drugs (NSAIDs), oral steroids, and braces will help decrease the inflammation and may alleviate the patient's symptoms. Intra-articular cortisone injections and physical therapy with modalities like phonophoresis can also be used to decrease the inflammation and pain at the subtalar joint.

RESULTS

Subtalar arthroscopy, overall, has excellent results. In a classic article, Williams and Ferkel demonstrated "86% good-to-excellent results" out of a subgroup of 29, each of which had pathology visualized on arthroscopy.[4] Perhaps the largest cohort, Ahn and colleagues reported a series of 115 patients, which included a range of subtalar pathologic conditions, with a mean follow-up period of 42 months. The mean American Orthopaedic Foot and Ankle Society (AOFAS) Ankle-Hindfoot Score in a cohort receiving subtalar arthroscopy increased from 69 points preoperatively to 89 points postoperatively. Ninety-seven percent of patients were satisfied with the surgical procedure.[5–7] More recently, Siddiqui and colleagues showed an improvement in AOFAS score from 49.6 to 75 at 6 months in a cohort of N = 6 patients.[1]

PROCEDURE

The patient is placed on the table in the supine position with an aggressive ipsilateral hip bump and the arthroscopy tower on the contralateral side of the position for ease of viewing. For posterior subtalar joint arthroscopy, the patient is placed in the prone position.[4]

It is important to mark the portals before insufflation to avoid losing the bony land-marks necessary for correct portal placement. The subtalar joint can be approached through several portals: lateral, accessory lateral, posteromedial, and posterolateral portals. The lateral and accessory lateral portals are easily developed by palpating into the sinus tarsi, anterior to the fibula, and posterior to the beak of the calcaneus.[8] When a posterior approach is used, the patient is in a prone position. The portals are made on the medial and lateral aspects of the Achilles tendon. A spinal needle is used over the skin to localize the superior-inferior aspects of the joint and introduced under fluoroscopy to ensure that posterior subtalar joint is entered as the proximity to the ankle joint allows for incorrect scope and instrument placement. In the supine approach, the anterolateral portal is the working portal and the lateral portal is the viewing portal (**Fig. 1**).

The most common complication of the procedure is damage to the surrounding neural structures. Tryfonidis and colleagues compared the distance from the sural nerve to the traditional portals for subtalar joint arthroscopy: anterior, middle, and posterior. The study concluded that the distances from the anterior, middle, and posterior portals to the nearest nerve were 21.3, 20.9, and 11.4 mm, respectively. Frey and colleagues evaluated the distance from the portals to the surrounding structures. The anterior portal was at an average distance of 17 mm from the dorsal intermediate cutaneous branch, 8 mm from a branch off the sural nerve, 21 mm from the peroneus tertius tendon but only 2 mm from a branch off the lesser saphenous vein. The posterior portal was at an average distance of 4 mm from the sural nerve, 11 mm from the peroneal tendons, and 15 mm from the Achilles tendon.[8] More recently, Lintz and colleagues performed a cadaveric study for structures at risk with a 4.0 mm arthroscope and a 3.5 mm shaver introduced through the anterior lateral and middle portals. The study was performed on 30 ft of 15 cadaveric bodies. The mean distance to a nerve from the portals was 4 mm. No nerve injury was appreciated. In three cases, a shaving lesion was appreciated on a peroneal tendon[9] (**Fig. 2**).

Once the subtalar joint is entered, the surgeon can perform an inspection of the intra-articular structures. Debridement of the joint is performed using sucker shavers, thermal ablation, and suction punches.[4]

PATHOLOGY

Sinus tarsi syndrome is the most distinctive diagnosis of the subtalar joint. Oloff and colleagues showed the high efficacy of subtalar joint arthroscopy in the diagnosis

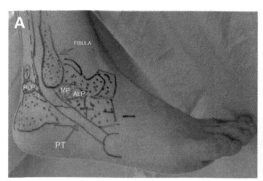
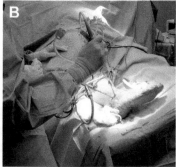

Fig. 1. (A, B) Landmarks for subtalar portal arthroscopy. ALP, anterolateral portal; MP, lateral portal; PLP, posterolateral portal; PT, peroneal tendons.

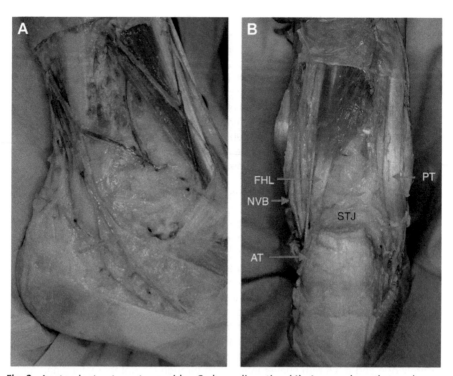

Fig. 2. Anatomic structures to consider. Cadaver dissection (*A*). Arrows show the sural nerve and posterior recurrent branch of sural nerve and its anatomic relations (*B*). AT, Achilles tendon; FHL, flexor hallucis longus tendon; NVB, neurovascular bundle; PT, peroneal tendons; STJ, subtalar joint position.

and treatment of sinus tarsi syndrome. In their study of 29 patients, 12 patients required 15 additional surgeries. Frey and colleagues reported on a subgroup of 14 ft with a pre-operative diagnosis of sinus tarsi syndrome. At the time of arthroscopy, all 14 diagnoses were revised. Ten patients were diagnosed with interosseous ligament tears, two with arthrofibrosis, and two with joint degeneration[4] (**Fig. 3**).

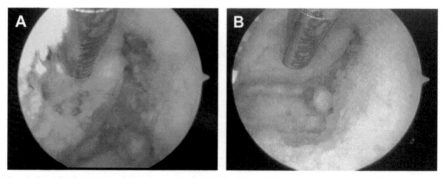

Fig. 3. (*A, B*) Thorough debridement of middle facet showing posterior inferior border of talonavicular joint (TNJ).

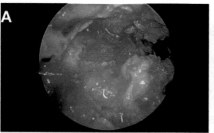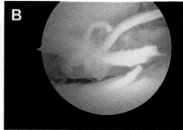

Fig. 4. (*A*) Arthroscopic curettage of middle facet; (*B*) Arthroscopic osteotome preparation of posterior facet.

More recently, Song and colleagues performed a retrospective review of 118 ankles having chronic lateral ankle instability with sinus tarsi pain who had undergone subtalar arthroscopy. They found that the rate of talocalcaneal interosseous ligament tears was 107/118 (90.7%). Interestingly, these same tears were only suspected in 81/118 (68.6%) on pre-operative MRI.[10,11] Lee showed that in 33 patients, pathology was found in 100% of patients symptomatic for sinus tarsi syndrome. In descending order, he reported a partial tear of the interosseous talo-calcaneal ligament (88%), synovitis (55%), partial tear of the cervical ligament (33%), and soft tissue impingement in (21%)[12,13] (**Fig. 4**).

There is a growing use for subtalar arthroscopy in the assistance of calcaneal fracture reduction. Arthroscopy of the subtalar joint to assist in the reduction and percutaneous fixation of intra-articular calcaneal fractures has also been described in the literature. In 2002, Gavlik and colleagues found that arthroscopy was able to detect incongruencies of the posterior facet in more than 25% of 47 intra-articular calcaneal fractures that appeared to be correctly reduced intraoperatively by fluoroscopy. The same authors reported that 22% of 59 intra-articular fractures were found to have a 1- to 2-mm step-off detected after visual and fluoroscopic evaluations of the reduction. More recently in 2017, Park and Yoon performed a comparative analysis for Sanders 2 calcaneal fractures.[14,15] In this study, 46 patients were treated for Sanders 2 calcaneal fractures with a sinus tarsi approach. Twenty-three patients were placed into a flourscopy only group and another 23 patients received intra-operative fluoroscopy and arthroscopy for fracture reduction. A post-op CT showed 73.9% reduction in the fluoroscopy only group compared to a 95.7% reduction in the fluoroscopy and arthroscopy group ($P = .04$).[14]

SUMMARY

Subtalar arthroscopy can be performed on a variety of different pathological conditions. It can be used as a strictly diagnostic modality as well as for various forms of reconstruction and fracture reduction. Although it is not used as commonly as ankle arthroscopy, there is a growing body of literature on its application as well as instructional technique in arthroscopy courses. Continued education and advancements in technology and instrumentation will only help to make this diagnostic and therapeutic modality more accessible to a growing body of foot and ankle surgeons. With these progressive developments, there will hopefully be an improvement in patient outcomes and a decrease in complication rates.

DISCLOSURES

J. Srour has nothing to disclose. L. Rubin is a consultant for Parcus and Vilex.

REFERENCES

1. Lee KB, Bai LB, Song EK, et al. Subtalar arthroscopy for sinus tarsi syndrome: arthroscopic findings and clinical outcomes of 33 consecutive cases. Journal of Arthroscopic & Related Surgery 2008;24(10):1130–4.
2. Park CH, Yoon DH. Role of subtalar arthroscopy in operative treatment of Sanders type 2 calcaneal fractures using a sinus tarsi approach. Foot Ankle Int 2018; 39(4):443–9.
3. Arshad Z, Bhatia M. Current concepts in sinus tarsi syndrome: a scoping review. Foot Ankle Surg 2020;27(6):615–21.
4. Gasparetto F, Collo G, Pisanu G, et al. Posterior ankle and subtalar arthroscopy: indications, technique, and results. Curr Rev Musculoskelet Med 2012;5(2): 164–70.
5. Song WT, Lee J, Lee JH, et al. A high rate of talocalcaneal interosseous ligament tears was found in chronic lateral ankle instability with sinus tarsi pain. Knee Surg Sports Traumatol Arthrosc 2021;29(11):3543–50.
6. Siddiqui MA, Chong KW, Yeo W, et al. Subtalar arthroscopy using a 2.4-mm zero-degree arthroscope: indication, technical experience, and results. Foot Ankle Spec 2010;3(4):167–71.
7. Whelan JH, Kiser C, Lazoritz JP, et al. Arthroscopic evaluation of the subtalar joint: a review and survey of pathology. J Am Podiatr Med Assoc 2019;111(2): Article_8.
8. Lopez-Ben R. Imaging of the subtalar joint. Foot Ankle Clin 2015;20(2):223–41.
9. Lintz F, Guillard C, Colin F, et al. Safety and efficiency of a 2-portal lateral approach to arthroscopic subtalar arthrodesis: a cadaveric study. Arthroscopy 2013;29(7):1217–23.
10. Lui TH, Tong SC. Subtalar arthroscopy: when, why and how? World J Orthop 2015;6(1):56–61.
11. Rubin LG. Subtalar joint arthroscopy. Clin Podiatr Med Surg 2011;28(3):539–50.
12. Perrera A, et al. Lateral hindfoot endoscopic Anterolateral/Posterolateral Subtalar arthrodesis: an effective minimally invasive technique to achieve subtalar fusion and deformity correction. Arthroscopy Techniques 2021;10(2):e423–9.
13. Muñoz G, Eckholt S. Subtalar arthroscopy: indications, technique and results. Foot Ankle Clin 2015;20(1):93–108.
14. Ahn JH, Lee SK, Kim YI, et al. Subtalar arthroscopic procedures for the treatment of subtalar pathologic conditions: 115 consecutive cases. Orthopedics 2009; 32(12):891.
15. Zaidi R, Hargunani R, calleja M, et al. MRI classification of subtalar joint osteoarthritis using a novel scoring system. Open J Radiol 2020;10(2).

Small Joint Arthroscopy of the Foot

Brian Derner, DPM, AACFAS[a],*, Richard Derner, DPM, FACFAS[b,1]

KEYWORDS

- Arthroscopy • Foot • Arthrodesis • Synovitis • Minimally invasive surgery

KEY POINTS

- Intimate knowledge of the arthroscopic anatomy is key for usage of these techniques.
- There is a very steep learning curve with extended surgical time and complication rate if procedures are not performed properly.
- Small joint arthroscopy has many applications and can be useful in the treatment of a wide array of joint pathologies.
- Arthroscopy can be performed as a joint-preserving option in lieu of joint-destructive procedures.

HISTORY

Arthroscopic treatment of the first metatarsophalangeal joint (MTPJ) was first described by Watanabe.[1] Bartlett first reported its use for osteochondral repairs in 1988.[2] Debnath and colleagues in 2006 noted 95% of patients remaining pain free at 2 years following the first MTPJ arthroscopy for treatment of early signs of degenerative joint disease.[3] Lui demonstrated a statistically significant correlation between joint cartilage erosion, joint synovitis, and pain in hallux valgus patients treated with arthroscopy of the first MTPJ.[4]

The use of arthroscopic technology for small joints of the foot have not been limited to the diagnosis and treatment of the first MTPJ pathology. Arthrodesis of the first tarsometatarsal (TMT) joint through a plantar-medial and dorsal-medial portal system has been recently described.[5] Lui in 2007 presented a TMT joint arthrodesis following a neglected fracture/dislocation through a 5-portal dorsal approach.[6] Parisien and Vangsness first reported the arthroscopic approach to subtalar joint (STJ) deformity in the literature in 1985,[7] but the calcaneocuboid and talonavicular joint (TNJ) resection for triple arthrodesis by arthroscopic means was also demonstrated by Lui in

---

[a] Kaiser San Leandro Medical Center, 2500 Merced Street, Suite 403, San Leandro, CA 94577, USA; [b] INOVA Fairfax Medical Center, Fairfax, VA, USA
[1] Present address: 6455 Lake Meadow Drive, Burke, VA 22015.
* Corresponding author.
E-mail address: brian.x.derner@kp.org

Clin Podiatr Med Surg 40 (2023) 445–457
https://doi.org/10.1016/j.cpm.2023.02.005
0891-8422/23/© 2023 Elsevier Inc. All rights reserved.

podiatric.theclinics.com

2006.[8] Bauer and colleagues in 2010 reported the first case of calcaneonavicular coalition resection by endoscopic means, resulting with an American Orthopedic Foot and Ankle Society (AOFAS) score of 82 at 2 years of follow-up.[9] Lesser MTPJ arthroscopy has also been described for plantar plate tears including evaluation and treatment of other lesser metatarsophalangeal (MTP) pathologies both in cadaveric specimens and human subjects. This technique described by Nery and colleagues[10,11] in 2014 has led to minimally invasive techniques for treatment of these pathologies.

Physical Examination and Diagnostic Modalities

Clinical examination of the range of motion should be initially evaluated. Clicking or crepitus needs to be carefully determined in the case of synovial impingement, meniscoid lesions, or an arthritic process. Inspection of the end range of motion should be determined to be of a painful or painless nature. Specific to the first MTPJ, a positive grind test should be evaluated for extensive osteochondral lesions.[12] Also, examination of the sesamoids with direct palpation and through range of motion is important in determining the cause of pain prior to proceeding with surgery specific to the first MTPJ. Hypermobility, typically of the first TMT joint, can also be noted and lead to discomfort for patients. Hypermobility can be tested by stabilizing the lateral forefoot in one hand, while gripping the first metatarsal neck in other and assessing sagittal and transverse plane motion.[13] In the case of a tarsal coalition, a peroneal spastic flatfoot along with immobility of the specific joint will be encountered. With lesser MTP pathology, care must be taken to evaluate for plantar plate rupture with a modified Lachman's test as well as full evaluation of intermetatarsal neuromas with a Mulder's click test. Most pathologies treated by small joint arthroscopy are related to either soft tissue or cartilage; however, there have been described cases of debridement of arthritic spurring with endoscopic techniques.

Along with a physical examination, radiographic evaluation must be performed. A combination of these modalities allows for most of the foot and ankle arthridities to be diagnosed. Weight-bearing anteroposterior (AP) and lateral radiographs can be very useful with diagnosing early-onset hallux rigidus (**Fig. 1**). The presence of joint space narrowing, periarticular osteophyte formation, and sesamoid hypertrophy on the AP radiograph aids in assessing the extent of disease in the joint. The extent of dorsal osteophyte formation noted on the lateral radiograph can assist the surgeon when deciding whether an arthroscopic or open treatment is indicated.[14–16]

However, in cases when the physical examination and radiographic results are not correlated, advanced imaging such as magnetic resonance imaging (MRI) or computed tomography are indicated (**Fig. 2**).[12] These are indicated in cases of trauma, soft tissue injuries, coalitions, or arthritis not visualized well on radiographs. MRI will help best with evaluation of cartilaginous pathology. Soft tissue pathology including capsular ligamentous laxity, scarring, or tearing can also be seen on MRI.

INDICATIONS

Careful evaluation and patient selection are paramount for any surgical intervention but may be even more so for arthroscopic versus open-type procedures. Patients suffering from impingement-type symptoms of various joints, hallux rigidus, midfoot trauma, inflammatory arthropathy, plantar plate tears, or osteochondral defects are candidates for small joint arthroscopic intervention. Resection of fibrous coalitions has been described as well endoscopically.[9] Patients who have wound-healing issues can also undergo minimally invasive joint preparation techniques for arthroscopy-assisted fusion of joints of the foot.

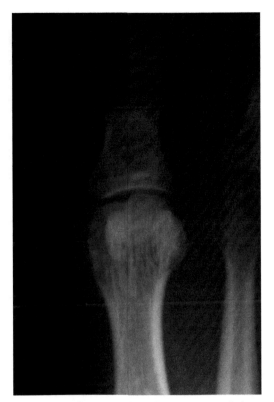

Fig. 1. Anteroposterior radiographic view of the first metatarsophalangeal joint with early-stage arthritis.

It is important to note there is a very steep learning curve in performing small joint arthroscopy. Knowledge of arthroscopic instrumentation, portal location, and superficial anatomy and possible injury to these structures must be understood. Therefore, open procedures may be indicated for patients with a difficult anatomy or pathology.[15,16]

FIRST METATARSOPHALANGEAL JOINT ARTHROSCOPY
Anatomy

The base of the proximal phalanx of the hallux is ovoid in shape; wider than it is tall; and concave both medial to lateral and dorsal to plantar. Little stability is gained from the chondroid nature of the first MTPJ due to the shallow surface for articulation between the phalanx and the metatarsal head.[13] The rounded head of the first metatarsal has a side-to-side curvature that is greater than the vertical curvature and is somewhat wider (20–24 mm) than its height (16–20 mm).[17] The articular surface, covered by hyaline cartilage, extends onto the dorsal aspect of the metatarsal head and continues plantarly into the medial and lateral grooves, which serve as articulations for the sesamoid bones, with the medial groove larger and deeper to accommodate for the larger tibial sesamoid. The plantar grooves are separated by a median crest, known as the crista.[17]

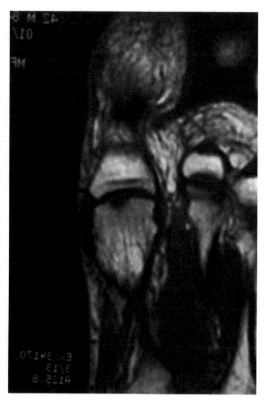

Fig. 2. MRI of the same joint with evidence of cartilaginous injury to the first metatarsal.

The joint capsule of the first metatarsal-phalangeal joint attaches close to cartilaginous edges dorsally; however, plantarly it attaches several millimeters proximal to the cartilage, with the plantar aspect of the capsule thicker than the dorsal aspect of the capsule due to the presence of the plantar MTP ligament. The metatarsosesamoid ligaments thicken the medial and lateral aspects of the joint capsule, along with the

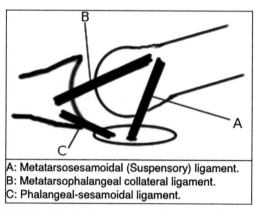

A: Metatarsosesamoidal (Suspensory) ligament.
B: Metatarsophalangeal collateral ligament.
C: Phalangeal-sesamoidal ligament.

Fig. 3. Anatomic depiction of the first metatarsophalangeal and sesamoidal joint complex.

medial and lateral collateral ligaments which tract from the medial and lateral metatarsal tubercles to the corresponding tubercles on the sides of the phalanx[17] (**Fig. 3**). The sesamoid bones of the flexor hallucis brevis muscle, which ossify between 10 and 12 years of age, are attached to the metatarsal via the metatarsosesamoidal ligaments and to the proximal phalanx of the hallux via the phalangeal-sesamoidal ligaments. The sesamoids are also firmly adhered to the plantar MTP ligament, which results in a firm attachment to the proximal phalanx. The sesamoids, therefore, do not move relative to the proximal phalanx, they move relative to the metatarsal.

Along with the ligamentous attachments described above, there are tendon attachments to the sesamoid bones as well. The tibial sesamoid provides an insertion point for the abductor hallucis, and the fibular sesamoid provides an insertion point for the adductor hallucis as well as the deep transverse metatarsal ligament. Contraction of the soft tissues that insert on the fibular sesamoid has been reported to contribute to the formation of hallux abductovalgus.[18]

Technique and Positioning

The patient is placed in the supine position upon the operating table, and the anesthesia department administers intravenous sedation. A sterile pneumatic ankle tourniquet is typically used and applied above the ankle. The great toe is distracted, and puckering at the joint confirms placement of the portals both dorsomedially and dorsolaterally (**Fig. 4**). A small incision is made longitudinally medial to the extensor hallucis longus (EHL) tendon. Blunt dissection is carried down to the joint to avoid any neurovascular injury, and the joint is then insufflated with approximately 5 mL of lactated Ringer's solution (**Fig. 5**). As the toe is distracted, a blunt obturator is placed into the dorsomedial portal and then into the joint. This is followed by the arthroscope. Most commonly, a 2.3-mm arthroscope with a 30° angulation is utilized for the first MPJ, which gives good visualization into the joint and allows for ease of movement within the joint. A second incision is then made lateral to the EHL tendon, and a needle is used initially for outflow. A mid-medial incision may be used to gain access to the plantar portion of the joint. This can aid in removing debris plantarly and evaluating lesions to the joint.

A blunt obturator is then used to enter the dorsolateral portal to allow for better egress of fluid and placement of instruments. The joint is then inspected, and a 2-mm probe is employed to evaluate the cartilage surface, look for lesions, and inspect the synovial recesses. A 1.9- to 2.0-mm shaver or thermocoagulator may be required to remove both hypertrophic and hemorrhagic synovitis within the joint including the

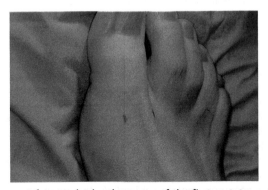

Fig. 4. Portal placement for standard arthroscopy of the first metatarsophalangeal joint.

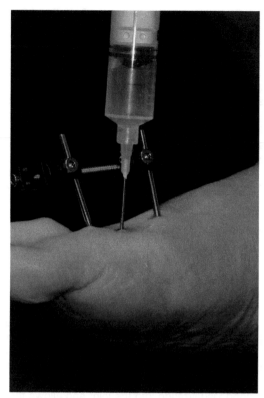

Fig. 5. Mini rail external fixator placement with insufflation of the joint to distract the joint for arthroscopy.

medial and plantar synovial proliferations. This will allow for better visualization within the joint.

Inspection of the joint proceeds in a clockwise pattern starting at the dorsal-central aspect of the metatarsal head, then laterally to the superior lateral surface, into the lateral gutter, the central aspect of the first metatarsal head, and then medially to the gutter and inferiorly to the tibial sesamoid-metatarsal joint. The proximal phalanx is then evaluated. The distal recesses medially and the articular surface of the base of the proximal phalanx and laterally are then evaluated. Siclari and Piras described a 10-point intra-articular examination of the joint.[19] Hull and colleagues further showed, in cadaveric specimens, 100% of the proximal phalanx base and an average of 57.5% of the first metatarsal head can be visualized via the standard dorsal portals.[20] They further noted other portals could be used for further evaluation of the first metatarsal head.[20] Nakajima also added two additional portal locations for visualization of the sesamoid apparatus.[21]

Traction is applied to the great toe either by an assistant or, if necessary, by a mini external fixator (**Fig. 6**). Although invasive, this latter technique gives excellent distraction of the great toe joint. Lastly, an articulating external fixator arm can give plantar-flexion at the same time as distraction to allow for easier evaluation of the plantar structures. The arthroscope is then placed into the dorsolateral portal to visualize the plantar fibular sesamoid-metatarsal joint. At this point, any obvious lesions are

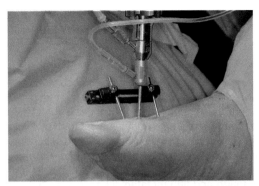

Fig. 6. Intraoperative image of the arthroscope in the distracted first metatarsophalangeal joint.

identified and removed via curettes creating sharp borders of cartilage. A piece of 0.035 Kirschner wire is then used to microfracture the subchondral bone plate. Meniscoid bodies that are identified are then removed with a small basket and cutters as necessary. Fibrous bands are also excised in a similar technique. Care should be taken plantarly to avoid injuring the sesamoid articulation and joint. Small joint-cutting blades and graspers, as well as a thermocoagulator, can be used in this second portal.

Outcomes of the First Metatarsophalangeal Joint Arthroscopy

In addition to noting increasing cartilage wear with worsening hallux valgus, Lui noted a statistically significant correlation between the size of cartilage defect and severity of hallux valgus using diagnostic arthroscopy of the first MTPJ.[4] Wang and colleagues in 2009 noted a statistically significant decrease in recurrence of acute gouty arthritis to the first MTPJ following arthroscopic debridement of tophi compared to patients treated by medical means alone.[22] Lui has also reported on performing arthroscopy on the great toe joint for hallux valgus deformity with good results.[4] He evaluated 94 feet treated for hallux valgus deformity and felt that arthroscopy was effective in improving both clinical and radiographic findings in patients with appropriate indications. These conditions included a reducible first intermetatarsal angle and no significant deformity to the distal first metatarsal articular angle. Patients were treated with an endoscopic soft tissue release, medial exostectomy; proximal screw placement after manual manipulation was performed to close the intermetatarsal angle. An endoscopic approach to soft tissue release at the first MTPJ for treatment of hallux valgus has also been reported with a significant increase in the AOFAS score at greater than 2 years of follow-up.[23] He also has described fusion of the first MTPJ for patients with severe bunion deformities.[24]

TARSOMETATARSAL JOINT ARTHROSCOPY
Anatomy

The first metatarsal-cuneiform joint (MCJ) is the largest of the TMT joints. The outline of the facets of the first MCJ is reniform in shape with the hilus laterally. The articular surface of the base of the first metatarsal is 25- to 30-mm deep and 16- to 20-mm wide, and the surface is concave dorsally and flat or slightly convex in the more plantar aspect of the joint.[25] The corresponding dorsal part of the distal aspect of the medial cuneiform is slightly convex, with the plantar aspect flat or slightly concave, allowing for inversion and eversion along the long axis of the metatarsal.

Portal Placement and Outcomes

Very little has been written on TMT joint arthroscopy. Lui and colleagues has described the fusion of the first MCJ after Lisfranc fracture dislocation.[5] Five portals were used to visualize these joints; medially for the first MCJ, between the first and second metatarsals and medial cuneiform; the second TMT joint is accessed via a portal at the junction of the central cuneiform bone and second and third metatarsals; the third and fourth metatarsal-tarsal joints are visualized via a portal between these bones and the lateral cuneiform and cuboid bone; and the fifth portal is at the junction of the Cuboid and fourth and fifth metatarsal bases (**Fig. 7**). Lui and colleagues also noted because fusion of the lateral column is rarely performed, tendon arthroplasty could be undertaken.[5]

There is a paucity of literature regarding this technique; however, minimizing dissection and preserving vascular supply have a definite benefit for arthrodesis. This advantage has been quite frequently identified when fusing the ankle arthroscopically.[26,27] One must be very skilled to identify and gain access to these joints arthroscopically because there is usually a large degree of osteophytic lipping and joint space narrowing.

Arthroscopic fusion alone of the first MCJ can be performed for hallux valgus or end-stage arthrosis. Two portals are used: one, dorsomedial, and the other, plantarmedial. Lui and colleagues used a 2.7-mm scope 30° and resected the joint with an osteotome and by microfracturing the subchondral bone.[5] He felt the advantage was better visualization, less shortening, better cosmetic result, and less postoperative pain over the open technique.

Recently, Liu and colleagues described the use of arthroscopy of the lateral-column TMT joints (fourth and fifth TMT joints) for treatment of pain and pathology of this complex in 24 patients.[28] They showed that 68.9% of joints had radiographic evidence of arthritis, but arthrofibrosis and chronic synovitis were seen in 87.5% and 75% of joints, respectively. Therefore, arthroscopic debridement of these joints is another joint sparing treatment option for lateral column arthrosis.[28]

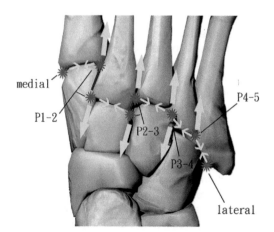

Fig. 7. Description of tarsometatarsal arthroscopic portal placement by Lui and Yuen.[15]

LESSER METATARSOPHALANGEAL JOINT ARTHROSCOPY
Anatomy and Portal Placement

The heads of the second through fifth metatarsals are convex and articulate with the concave proximal phalanx bases. The MTPJ capsule attaches in a groove adjacent to the articular surface. The collateral as well as the accessory collateral ligaments of that joint are attached to the metatarsal tubercles at the heads, proximal to the articular cartilage. The plantar MTPJ ligament also known as the plantar plate attaches the metatarsal head to the plantar proximal phalanx base.[16]

Positioning of the foot is identical to the first MTPJ arthroscopy, and portal placement is very similar to the first MTPJ with dorsomedial and dorsolateral portals on either side of the long extensor tendon at the level of the lesser MTPJ. The dorsal digital branch of the deep peroneal nerve runs medially on the second MTPJ, and care must be taken to avoid this structure with this procedure. Manual traction can be used for distraction of the joint during lesser MTPJ arthroscopy.[10] In addition, a 2.7- or 1.9-mm arthroscope can be used for visualization of the joint. Nery and colleagues[10] showed a 96% overall accuracy of evaluation of the entire lesser MTP joint complex via this technique.

Treatments

Arthroscopy is a very helpful adjunct in these small joints to allow for visualization and debridement of arthrofibrosis or synovitis on patients with recalcitrant pain following conservative management. Lui and Yuen have described treatment of plantar plate tearing from an all-inside arthroscopic approach using suture materials.[15,29] In addition, he described a tendon arthroplasty technique for the treatment of Freiberg's infarction with utilization of an accessory portal for insertion of the extensor digitorum brevis tendon, fashioned with suture.[15,29]

CHOPART JOINT ARTHROSCOPY (TALONAVICULAR AND CALCANEOCUBOID JOINT)
Anatomy

The midtarsal joint is comprised of the TNJ and the calcaneocuboid joint (CCJ). The TNJ is condylar in nature, while the CCJ is a saddle joint. These joints cannot act independently, as motion in the STJ and CCJ is required for motion in the TNJ. The head of the talus is convex in all directions and bears at least three recognizable articular areas: an ovoid area for articulation with the navicular, a triangular facet for the plantar calcaneonavicular ligament, and a long oval area plantarly for the anterior calcaneal articular facet. The posterior surface of the navicular is ovoid in shape and broader laterally than medially; the articular surface is concave and wholly articular with the head of the talus. The talonavicular ligament is a wide, thin band that connects the superior surface of the talar neck to the dorsal surface of the navicular. The calcaneonavicular ligament component of the bifurcate ligament also serves to provide medial support to the CCJ and lateral support to the TNJ. The anterior surface of the calcaneus is roughly shaped like an inverted triangle. The articular surface is concave from superior to inferior and convex transversely, giving the characteristic saddle shape. The posterior surface of the cuboid has a saddle shape corresponding to the anterior surface of the calcaneus.[17]

Talonavicular Joint Arthroscopy

For TNJ arthroscopy, portals are placed at the level of the TNJ. Originally, Oloff and colleagues described medial, central, and lateral portals.[30] The medial portal is placed superior to the tibialis posterior tendon, the central portal is placed just medial to the tibialis anterior (TA) tendon, and the lateral portal is just medial to the EHL.[30] Hammond and colleagues described a dorsomedial portal, just lateral to the TA tendon, and a dorsolateral portal.[31] This portal was found by inverting the foot and palpating the lateral talar head at the joint line.[31] The modified dorsolateral portal was just medial to the EHL tendon, described by Ross and colleagues.[32] Their study showed an average distance of 0.9 mm to the neurovascular bundle when making this new dorsolateral approach. They also showed the saphenous nerve was 6.8 mm inferior to the TA tendon, so the portal must be directly medial to the TA.[32] Xavier and colleagues also showed safety in cadaveric models for all these portal sites and showed that only 5.3% of these four portals showed possible neurovascular compromise.[33] Therefore, there is low risk associated, and these procedures are feasible for treatment of TNJ pathology including synovitis, osteochondral defects, osteoarthritis, or other inflammatory arthropathies.[33] A pin distractor medially can aid in distraction of the joint along with insufflation of the lactated Ringer's solution.

Hammond and colleagues studied TNJ arthroscopy for fusion of the joint.[31] They were able to visualize 98.6% of the navicular and 83.2% of the talus in the TNJ for joint preparation. However, they were 1 mm from the lateral branch of the deep peroneal nerve, and this could lead to possible neurologic complications. In addition, this was a joint destructive arthroscopy and, therefore, could overestimate the visualization of the TNJ in arthroscopic debridements of synovitis.[31] Ross and colleagues performed a case series with three TNJ arthroscopy patients treated by microfracture of osteochondral lesions.[32] These patients all had improvements in their outcomes measures, and repeat MRIs showed reparative fibrocartilage in all patients.[32] Other studies of osteochondral lesions of the TNJ have showed positive outcomes with microfracture in the instance of a kissing osteochondral lesion of the talus and navicular.[34] Capsular release of the TNJ has also been described for patients with arthrofibrosis after a talar neck fracture.[35]

Calcaneocuboid Joint Arthroscopy

Oloff and colleagues also described the portal for CCJ arthroscopy.[30] The superior portal was placed at the level of the anterior process of the calcaneus, and the inferior portal is directly inferior to this, roughly 2-3 cm, but superior to the peroneus brevis tendon[30] (**Fig. 8**). Very little evidence-based studies have been described for CCJ arthroscopy and pathology. Indications for arthroscopic treatment of CCJ pathology

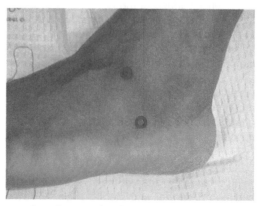

Fig. 8. Portal placement for calcaneocuboid joint arthroscopy (*red circles*).

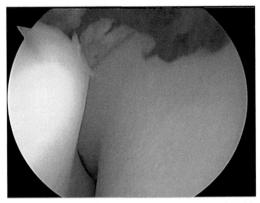

Fig. 9. Intraoperative image of the calcaneocuboid joint with synovitis present.

include loose bodies, osteochondritis dissecans, osteophytes, synovial impingement, infection, biopsy, or inflammatory synovitis (**Fig. 9**).

Oloff and colleagues had 6 patients who underwent CCJ arthroscopy with positive results.[30] However, 33.3% of patients had some type of peroneal tendinitis or peroneal fibrosis after surgical treatment of their CCJ pathology.[30] Lui also described a technique for "refreshment" of a nonunion site of a CCJ distraction arthrodesis nonunion, which involved implementation of cancellous bone grafting with positive fusion at 12 weeks (without any change in hardware).[36]

Postoperative Course

Portal sites are usually closed with nonabsorbable suture in a simple or horizontal mattress fashion. A petroleum-based dressing is applied with 4 × 4 and soft dressing. Patients are put into a controlled ankle motion boot for 1-2 weeks until sutures are removed in the cases of simple debridements and synovectomies. Patients who undergo fusion procedures arthroscopically or osteochondral lesion repairs are immobilized in a posterior splint in the immediate postoperative period. It is ultimately up to the discretion of the surgeon on when best to weight-bear their patients after these types of procedures. Most likely, patients who undergo fusions will have radiographic evidence of bony trabeculation across the fusion site prior to weight-bearing.

Complications

Depending on the arthroscopic location, there can be anatomical injuries to the nearby structures. Careful portal placement is paramount for mitigating excess risk to these surgeries. Infection, neurovascular injury, cartilage injury or damage from shaving, wound-healing problems, fibrosis of nearby tendinous structures, hematoma, seroma, decreased range of motion, scarring, and stiffness are all potential complications. Sterile technique, blunt dissection, appropriate portal placement, and prior training in these techniques all improve outcomes. Overzealous debridement can also lead to worsening arthrosis of the joint.

SUMMARY

Overall, small joint arthroscopy gained a slow increase in popularity for specific pathological issues. The combination of learning curve, surgical time, and specific indications has stunted its overall acceptance. Despite this, there is a definite benefit to this technique in both diagnosis and management of small joint pathology. Understanding the nuances of anatomy, arthroscopic instrumentation, distraction of joints, and potential hazards during surgery will often provide a gratifying result for the patient.

DISCLOSURE

There authors have nothing to disclose.

REFERENCES

1. Watanabe M. Selfox-arthroscope. In: Watanabe no. 24 arthroscope (monograph). Tokyo: Teishin Hospital; 1972. p. 46–53.
2. Bartlett DH. Arthroscopic management of osteochondritis dissecans. Arthroscopy 1988;4(1):51–4.
3. Debnath UK, Hemmady MV, Hariharan K. Indications for and technique of first MTP arthroscopy. Foot Ankle Int 2006;27(12):1049–54.
4. Lui TH. First metatarsophalangeal joint arthroscopy in patients with hallux valgus. Arthroscopy 2008;24(10):1122–9.
5. Lui TH, Chan KB, Ng S. Arthroscopic lapidus arthrodesis. Arthroscopy 2005; 21(12):1516.e1–4.
6. Lui TH. Arthroscopic tarsometatarsal (Lisfranc) arthrodesis. Knee Surg Sports Traumatol Arthrosc 2007;25:671–5.
7. Parisien JS, Vangsness T. Arthroscopy of the subtalar joint: an experimental approach. Arthroscopy 1985;1:53–7.
8. Lui TH. New technique of arthroscopic triple arthrodesis. Arthroscopy 2006;22(4): 464.e1–5.
9. Bauer T, Golano P, Hardy P. Endoscopic resection of a calcaneonavicular coalition. Knee Surg Sports Traumatol Arthrosc 2010;18:669–72.
10. Nery C, Coughlin MJ, Baumfeld D, et al. Lesser metatarsal phalangeal joint arthroscopy: anatomic description and comparative dissection. Arthroscopy 2014;30(8):971–9.
11. Nery C, Baumfeld T, Raduan F, et al. Flexor to extensor tendon transfer and weil osteotomy to treat grade IV plantar plate tears. Tech Foot Ankle Surg 2018; 19(2):84–8.
12. Shurnas PS, Coughlin MJ. Arthritic conditions of the foot. In: Coughlin MJ, Mann RA, Saltzman CL, editors. Surgery of the foot and ankle. Vol 1. 8th ed. Philadelphia, PA: Mosby Elsevier; 2007. p. 867–906.
13. Carreira DS. Arthroscopy of the hallux. Foot Ankle Clin N Am 2009;14:105–14.
14. Derner R, Naldo J. Small joint arthroscopy of the foot. Clin Podiatr Med Surg 2011;28(3):551–60.
15. Lui TH, Yuen CP. Small joint arthroscopy in foot and ankle. Foot Ankle Clin 2015; 20(1):123–38.
16. Reeves CL, Shane AM, Payne T, et al. Small joint arthroscopy in the foot. Clin Podiatr Med Surg 2016;33(4):565–80.
17. Hirsch B.E. and Minugh-Purvis N., Anatomy of the Lower Extremity, Pennsylvania College of Podiatric Medicine, 1993, Philadelphia.
18. McBride ED. The McBride bunion hallux valgus operation: refinements in the successive surgical steps of the operation. J Bone Joint Surg Am 1967;49(8): 1675–83.
19. Siclari A, Piras M. Hallux metatarsophalangeal arthroscopy: indications and techniques. Foot Ankle Clin 2015;20:109–22.

20. Hull M, Campbell JT, Jeng CL, et al. Measuring Visualized joint surface in hallux metatarsophalangeal arthroscopy. Foot Ankle Int 2018;39(8):978–83.

21. Nakajima K. Arthroscopy of the first metatarsophalangeal joint. J Foot Ankle Surg 2018;57(2):357–63.

22. Wang CC, Lien SB, Huang GS, et al. Arthroscopic elimination of monosodium urate deposition of the first metatarsophalangeal joint reduces the recurrence of gout. Arthroscopy 2009;25(2):153–8.

23. Lui TH, Chan KB, Chan LK. Endoscopic distal soft-tissue release in the treatment of hallux valgus: a cadaveric study. Arthroscopy 2010;26(8):1111–6.

24. Lui TH. Arthroscopic arthrodesis of the first metatarsophalangeal joint in hallux valgus deformity. Arthroscopy Techniques 2017;6(5):e1481–7.

25. Glick JM, Ferkel RD. Arthroscopic ankle arthrodesis. In: Ferkel RD, editor. The foot & ankle. Philadelphia, PA: Lippincott-Raven; 1996. p. 215–29.

26. Glick JM, Morgan CD, Myerson MS, et al. Ankle arthrodesis using an arthroscopic method: long-term follow-up of 34 cases. Arthroscopy 1996;12(4):428–34.

27. Faure C. The skeleton of the anterior foot. Anat Clin 1981;3:49–65.

28. Liu GT, Vanpelt MD, Manchanda K, et al. Arthroscopic findings in refractory symptomatic fourth and fifth tarsometatarsal joints. J Foot Ankle Surg 2022. https://doi.org/10.1053/j.jfas.2022.02.009.

29. Lui TH. Arthroscopic interpositional arthroplasty of the second metatarsophalangeal joint. Arthroscopy Techniques 2016;5(6):e1333–8.

30. Oloff L, Schulhofer SD, Fanton G, et al. Arthroscopy of the calcaneocuboid and talonavicular joints. J Foot Ankle Surg 1996;35(2):101–8.

31. Hammond AW, Phisitkul P, Femino J, et al. Arthroscopic debridement of the talonavicular joint using dorsomedial and dorsolateral portals: a cadaveric study of safety and access. Arthroscopy 2011;27(2):228–34.

32. Ross KA, Seaworth CM, Smyth NA, et al. Talonavicular arthroscopy for osteochondral lesions. Foot Ankle Int 2014;35(9):909–15.

33. Xavier G, Oliva XM, Rotinen M, et al. Talonavicular joint arthroscopic portals: a cadaveric study of feasibility and safety. Foot Ankle Surg 2016;22(3):205–9.

34. Wan YTO, Lui TH. Arthroscopic debridement and microfracture of osteochondral lesion of the talar head. Arthroscopy Techniques 2019;8(9):e969–73.

35. Lui TH. Arthroscopic capsular release of the talocalcaneonavicular joint. Arthroscopy Techniques 2016;5(6):e1305–9.

36. Lui TH. Arthroscopic revision of nonunion of calcaneocuboid distraction arthrodesis. Foot 2013;23(4):172–5.

Arthroscopic Ankle Arthrodesis

Michael S. Lee, DPM, FACFAS[a],*, Samantha M. Figas, DPM, AACFAS[b],
Jordan P. Grossman, DPM, FACFAS[b]

KEYWORDS

• Ankle • Arthritis • Ankle arthrodesis • Ankle arthroscopy

KEY POINTS

• Arthroscopic arthrodesis of the ankle provides faster time to union with decrease complication rates.
• Arthroscopic ankle arthrodesis has become easier with advancements in surgical technique and instrumentations.
• Ankle arthrodesis remains the gold standard for end-stage ankle arthritis.

Despite the increasing popularity of TAR, ankle arthrodesis remains the gold standard for the treatment of end-stage ankle arthritis.[1,2] Historically, open techniques have been utilized for ankle arthrodesis. There have been many variations and techniques described, including transfibular, anterior, medial, and miniarthrotomy.[3–17] Inherent disadvantages to these open techniques include postoperative pain, delayed or nonunion, wound complications, shortening, prolonged healing times, and prolonged hospital stays.[18–20]

Arthroscopic ankle arthrodesis provides the foot and ankle surgeon with an alternative to the traditional open techniques. Arthroscopic ankle arthrodesis has demonstrated faster union rates, decreased complications, reduced postoperative pain, and shorter hospital stays.[3,20–31] Although once considered technically difficult, advancements in techniques and instrumentation have flattened the learning curve once encountered with the arthroscopic technique.

Schneider first reported arthroscopic ankle arthrodesis in 1983 and reported faster time to union, earlier mobilization, and reduced patient morbidity.[32] More recent studies have demonstrated similar results with faster union rates, fewer complications, and shorter hospital stays.[3,21–23,29–31] This article will discuss the indications, technique, and complications associated with arthroscopic ankle arthrodesis.

---

[a] Capital Orthopaedics & Sports Medicine, 12499 University Avenue, Suite 210, Clive, IA 50325, USA; [b] Cleveland Clinic, Akron Greneral, Akron, OH 44307, USA
* Corresponding author.
E-mail address: mlee@dsmcapitalortho.com

Clin Podiatr Med Surg 40 (2023) 459–470
https://doi.org/10.1016/j.cpm.2023.02.001
0891-8422/23/© 2023 Elsevier Inc. All rights reserved.

podiatric.theclinics.com

INDICATIONS/CONTRAINDICATIONS

Arthroscopic ankle arthrodesis may be indicated in patients with end-stage arthritis due to a variety of causes, including rheumatoid arthritis, posttraumatic arthritis, arthrogryposis, septic arthritis, inflammatory arthritis, avascular necrosis of the talus, idiopathic osteoarthritis, and chronic ankle instability. The most frequently encountered cause, however, remains posttraumatic arthritis.[21]

The primary indication for ankle arthrodesis is persistent pain in the arthritic ankle joint that has not responded to conservative treatments, including analgesics, nonsteroidal anti-inflammatory drugs, corticosteroid injections, and orthoses or bracing for several months.[3,22,28] Although not currently Food and Drug Administration-approved for the ankle joint, hyaluronic acid injections may also be utilized before proceeding with arthrodesis or replacement. A study by Salk, Chang and colleagues[33] showed promising results of using sodium hyaluronate injections for ankle arthritis because they demonstrated significant pain relief and improved function following a series of these injections. Platelet-rich plasma injections are becoming more popular for patients with arthritis who have failed all other conservative therapy seeking to avoid surgical intervention. More recent studies have shown benefit in knee arthritis; however, current studies are not supporting the same benefit in the ankle.[34,35]

Limitations of arthroscopic ankle arthrodesis are typically related to deformity or malalignment of the ankle joint. Various studies have indicated that malalignment greater than 10° to 15° will make reduction of the ankle joint and deformity difficult.[23,36] Ferkel and Hewitt indicated that patients with significant ankle deformity, either significant varus or valgus, are better suited for an open technique while those that require arthrodesis in situ are better suited for the arthroscopic technique.[27] Tang and colleagues[37] stated that arthroscopy should not be advised when a large ankle deformity is present. However, a study done in 2007 by Gougoulias and colleagues[26] showed that patients with marked deformity of greater than 10° to 15° of varus or valgus can be treated effectively using arthroscopy, depending on surgeon experience. This has been supported by a more recent study by Issac and colleagues[38] in 2021, which showed similar postoperative alignment and union rates when comparing open versus arthroscopic ankle arthrodesis in coronal plane deformities greater than 15°. In 2017, Schmid and colleagues[39] demonstrated equivalent postoperative radiographic alignment between open and arthroscopic ankle arthrodesis with both minimal and severe preoperative coronal plane deformities. These authors discussed how arthroscopic ankle arthrodesis can be performed in coronal plane deformities up to 25°.[39] The main factor in this study was open technique was chosen over arthroscopic specifically with greater tibial deformities than ankle joint deformities, with arthroscopic only addressing tibial plafond angles of 0° to 19° where open could address deformities 40° or higher.[39] As surgeons surpass the previous believed limits of arthroscopy, there currently is no consensus on the maximum degree of deformity that can be addressed in an arthroscopic ankle arthrodesis.

Other contraindications of arthroscopic ankle arthrodesis should also be noted, including excessive bone loss, neuropathic joints, active infections, and poor bone stock.[22] Avascular necrosis of the talus may also be a contraindication.

SURGICAL TECHNIQUE

Arthroscopic ankle arthrodesis is performed under general or spinal anesthesia. A thigh tourniquet is typically used for hemostasis and the leg is prepped to the tibial tuberosity. A bump under the ipsilateral hip is used to slightly internally rotate the leg.

The ankle is insulflated with approximately 20 mL of normal sterile saline using an 18-gauge needle. Standard anteromedial and anterolateral portals are utilized. A 2.7°mm, 30° arthroscope is then introduced into the ankle joint. The author prefers to use large joint power shavers and burrs while using a 2.7-mm arthroscope rather than the 4.0-mm arthroscope. A noninvasive ankle distractor is applied to the ankle to allow for complete visualization from anterior to posterior, as well as both the medial and lateral gutters (**Fig. 1**).

A 3.85-mm full radius incisor blade is used to aggressively debride the anterior joint of any hypertrophic synovium, fibrosis, or loose bodies. In some cases, aggressive resection of anterior tibiotalar osteophytes is required for proper joint visualization. A curette is inserted to aggressively remove any remaining articular cartilage (**Fig. 2**). A grasping forcep or resector may be used to remove the cartilage fragments that typically collect in the posterior aspect of the joint (**Fig. 3**). A 4.0-mm full radius burr or 4.85-mm acromion burr is then used to resect the subchondral plate (**Fig. 4**). A curved osteotome is then used to fish scale the subchondral plates of both the tibia and talus (**Fig. 5**). Ideally, healthy bleeding bone will be visualized throughout the tibiotalar articulation (**Fig. 6**). Similar preparation is often completed in the distal portion of the distal syndesmotic space as well. The joint is then irrigated and all loose bodies or fragments are evacuated.

All arthroscopic instrumentation is then removed from the ankle joint. Platelet-rich plasma or other bone graft substitutes may then be inserted into the ankle joint at the surgeon's discretion. The noninvasive distractor is removed from the foot. Proper bony apposition is confirmed using fluoroscopy. Care is also taken to confirm proper positioning clinically.

Fixation is achieved with 2 or 3 large-diameter cannulated screws. Typically, the preferred technique is to place 2 stacked screws from the medial tibia into the talar body (1 directed slightly posterior and 1 slightly anterior) and a third screw from the fibula across the syndesmosis into the tibia then across the ankle joint into the medial talar dome (**Fig. 7**).

The portals and stab incisions for screw placement are closed with simple sutures. The extremity is placed in a controlled ankle motion (CAM) boot. In most cases, the patient is discharged to home the day of surgery. Sutures are removed at 1 week postoperatively, and the patient is placed in a below-the-knee cast. Strict adherence to nonweight-bearing is followed for 6 to 7 weeks. Weight-bearing is then advanced

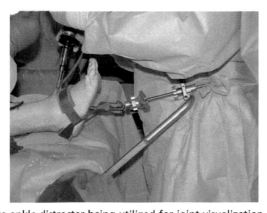

Fig. 1. Noninvasive ankle distracter being utilized for joint visualization.

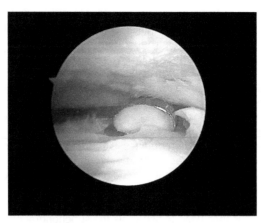

Fig. 2. Curettage of the remaining articular surface.

based on radiographic healing and clinical symptoms in a CAM boot (**Fig 8**). Typically, at approximately 10 weeks postop, the patient is placed in a rocker-bottom sole shoe and ankle-foot-orthoses (AFO), and activities are advanced as tolerated. The AFO is continued for up to an additional 3 months and the rocker-bottom sole is continued according to the patient's preference.

DISCUSSION

Arthroscopic ankle arthrodesis has been well studied and has demonstrated favorable postoperative outcomes.[20–29] Advantages include decreased time to union, diminished postoperative pain, comparable union rates, shorter hospital stays, and earlier patient mobilization.[20–29,40–43] Preservation of the bony contour and the large amount of cancellous bony contact allow for significant stability and rigid internal fixation.[22,43] This is contradictory to the traditional open techniques that have often implemented planalresection decreasing bony contact and decreasing inherent stability. Additionally, "flat-topping" the talus and tibia makes proper positioning of the foot in the sagittal plane significantly more difficult because precise bone cuts are

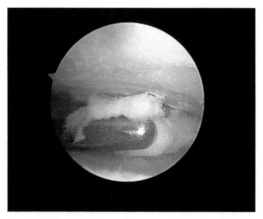

Fig. 3. Removal of the cartilage fragments after aggressive curettage.

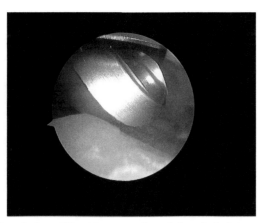

Fig. 4. Full radius burr being utilized to resect the subchondral plate.

required. O'Brian and colleagues[20] showed there was greater variability of ankle positions in patients that received the open ankle fusion compared with the arthroscopic technique.

Stetson and Ferkel recommended an open technique in ankles that have malrotation or anterior–posterior translation of the tibiotalar joint.[36] They also thought ankles that had a deformity of greater than 15° of varus or valgus should be treated with an open technique.[36] Gougoulias and colleagues,[26] however, achieved successful arthroscopic ankle arthrodeses on ankle deformities of 15° to 45° of varus or valgus. They point out that, although they were able to successfully fuse ankles with marked deformity, there is a significant learning curve associated with the procedure.[26] Other recent studies also suggest that it may be possible to arthroscopically fuse ankles with deformities of 25° or greater.[23,38,39] This author has found that malalignment of up to 15° is acceptable for arthroscopic arthrodesis. In some cases, particularly patients with severe valgus malalignment of the ankle, the joint may be reducible clinically. In these cases, arthroscopic ankle arthrodesis is possible but preoperative planning includes the possibility of converting to a miniarthrotomy.

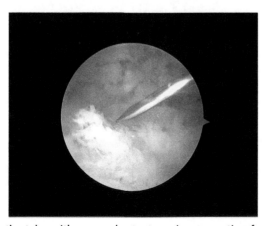

Fig. 5. Fish scaling the talus with a curved osteotome in preparation for arthrodesis.

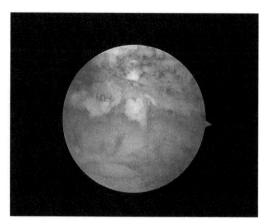

Fig. 6. Joint surfaces after preparation for arthrodesis.

Union may be described in 2 different ways: clinical union and radiographic union. Clinical union is described as having a stable, painless ankle joint. Radiographic union is defined as having bridging trabeculae between the tibia and the talus.[26,44]

Interestingly, nonunion rates between arthroscopic ankle arthrodesis and open techniques are similar. Collman and colleagues[22] reported a 93% clinical fusion rate and a 74% radiographic union rate, indicating a subset of arthroscopic ankle arthrodesis cases that have a clinical union rate of 87.2%. A nonunion rate of 7.6% was reported by Winson and colleagues[23] in their review of 118 arthroscopic ankle fusions. Similar union rates in other studies have been reported with a range from 73% to 100%.[3,17,20,27–31,40,42,45–47]

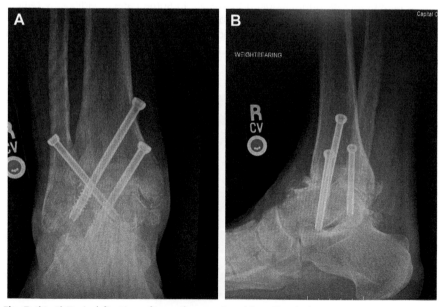

Fig. 7. (*A, B*) Typical fixation after arthroscopic ankle arthrodesis.

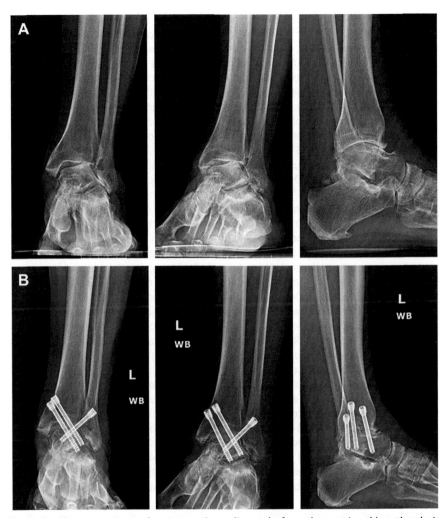

Fig. 8. (*A*, *B*) Preoperative and postoperative radiographs for arthroscopic ankle arthrodesis.

The negative effects cigarette smoking has on both soft-tissue and bone healing have been well documented.[48–53] The role of nicotine in ankle arthrodesis nonunions has also been well documented and may present a relative risk of nonunion 4 times that seen in nonsmokers.[18,54] Arthroscopic ankle fusions had not shown this similar trend and theorized that the ill-effects of smoking are countered by the minimally invasive approach.[22,55] However, more recent study by Issac and colleagues[38] demonstrated 10 times higher nonunion rate in smokers regardless to their preoperative deformity or operative technique.

Studies demonstrating union rates correlated to patient comorbidities have been limited primarily to rheumatoid arthritis.[46,49,50] Other variables, such as a history of arthritis etiology, effects of bone graft substitutes, body mass index (BMI), and preexisting deformity, have not been extensively studied with regards to arthroscopic ankle arthrodesis. In one study, 4 of 5 patients with posttraumatic arthritis developed nonunions.[22] The higher concentration of sclerotic bone adjacent to the subchondral plate may contribute to this increased incidence of nonunion, reinforcing the importance of aggressive joint resection.[29,40,56,57] A more recent study by Berk and colleagues[30] demonstrated comparable, if not higher, union rates with arthroscopic arthrodesis versus open in postop traumatic ankle arthritis. In this study, 6/24 open technique required revision surgery for a nonunion while arthroscopic technique had 1 out of 11 patients.[30] Overall, definitive union rate was achieved in 22 out of 23 open arthrodeses and 11 out of 11 arthroscopic arthrodesis.[30] Malalignment of the ankle may also predispose to nonunion of the arthroscopic ankle arthrodesis.[22] Issac and colleagues[38] demonstrated similar union rates between open and arthroscopic techniques with greater than 15° of coronal plane deformity.

A clear advantage of the use of arthroscopic arthrodesis over open techniques is the time to fusion is reduced. Open ankle fusions have a reported average fusion time of approximately 14 weeks.[30,40,41,48] In a study of 39 arthroscopic arthrodeses, Collman and colleagues[22] reported an average fusion time of 47 days, whereas Glick and colleagues[42] noted a 9-week average fusion time in 34 ankles. Other studies have noted time to fusion for arthroscopic ankle arthrodesis from 8.9 to 12 weeks.[3,23,29,30,48] One theory to support the decreased fusion time is that the arthroscopic technique does not disrupt the periarticular blood supply facilitating healing.[29,40,42,49]

Honnenahalli Chandrappa performed a meta-analysis of the literature in 2017, which demonstrated decreased length of stay with arthroscopic ankle arthrodesis.[58,59] Within this systematic review, included studies were those of O'Brien and colleagues[20] who demonstrated that patients who underwent arthroscopic arthrodesis had hospital stays of 1.6 days, versus the open techniques that averaged 3.4 days in the hospital. Other studies have also supported these findings. Ogilvie-Harris and colleagues[28] reported an average discharge from the hospital of 1 day. Dent and colleagues[25] also reports an average stay of less than 2 days. Cameron and Ulrich also reported on outpatient arthroscopic ankle arthrodesis.[3] In another study of 39 patients, only 3 were not discharged the day of the procedure.[22] Zvijc and colleagues[29] reported an average hospitalization of 3 days for those who had an open procedure as compared with 1 day for those who received an arthroscopic arthrodesis. Pain levels within this study were much less then expected in the arthroscopic group, which lead to more arthroscopic ankle arthrodesis to be performed on an outpatient basis.[29] In yet another study, arthroscopic fusion compared with open techniques demonstrated significant cost savings.[60]

Arthroscopic ankle arthrodesis has demonstrated reduced pain postoperatively as well as a shorter reliance on pain medication.[25,28,29,31] This author has also noted a significant decrease in postoperative pain with the arthroscopic technique. It is now common practice for arthroscopic ankle arthrodeses to be performed in outpatient surgery centers, with the decision to admit a patient postoperatively determined by their comorbidities and not postoperative pain concerns.

Other advantages of arthroscopic arthrodesis, include decreased blood loss, less disruption of the soft tissue structures around the ankle, and diminished risk of thrombosis due to shorter immobilization times. Multiple studies have also noted reduced tourniquet time.[20,60–62] There is also minimal loss of length of the lower limb, as well as minimal clinical deformity or shape changes to the ankle.[25]

Arthroscopic ankle arthrodesis may be preferred to an open technique in at-risk patients.[22,34,63] The earlier mobilization due to a shorter time to union is beneficial in patients with rheumatoid arthritis, advanced age, diabetes, and other autoimmune diseases.[40,47] The senior author has utilized the arthroscopic technique in these at-risk patients with great success but cautions its use in patients with peripheral neuropathy.

Finally with the ever-growing popularity of TAR, there are more recent studies comparing clinical outcomes of TAR to both open and arthroscopic ankle arthrodesis. In a recent study by Veljkovic and colleagues,[64] comparable clinical outcomes of TAR, arthroscopic ankle arthrodesis, and open ankle arthrodesis were noted. The authors did observe higher reoperation rates in TARs, which included procedures such as gutter debridements, ligament repairs, poly exchange, and cyst debridements.[64]

SUMMARY

Arthroscopic ankle arthrodesis provides the foot and ankle surgeon with an alternative to traditional open techniques. Advancements in arthroscopic techniques and instrumentation have made the procedure easier to perform. Arthroscopic ankle arthrodesis has demonstrated faster rates of union, decreased complications, reduced postoperative pain, and shorter hospital stays.[3,20–31] Adherence to sound surgical techniques, particularly with regards to joint preparation, is critical for success. Comorbidities, such as increased BMI, a history of smoking, malalignment, and posttraumatic arthritis, should be carefully considered when contemplating arthroscopic ankle arthrodesis. However, more recent studies have demonstrated improved results when treating patients with posttraumatic arthritis or those with malalignment.[30,38,39] Although TAR continues to increase in popularity over open ankle arthrodesis, recent studies have demonstrated arthroscopic ankle arthrodesis remains a viable alternative for the management of the end-stage arthritic ankle.[64]

REFERENCES

1. Coester LM, Saltman CL, Leapold J, et al. Long-term results following ankle arthrodesis for post-traumatic arthritis. J Bone Joint Surg 2001;83:219–28.
2. Buck P, Morrey BF, Chao EY. The optimum position of arthrodesis of the ankle. J Bone Joint Surg 1987;69:1052–62.
3. Cameron SE, Ulrich P. Arthroscopic arthrodesis of the ankle joint. Arthroscopy 2000;16:21–6.
4. Cheng YM, Chen SK, Chen JC, et al. Revision of ankle arthrodesis. Foot Ankle Int 2003;24:321–5.
5. Colgrove RC, Bruffey JD. Ankle arthrodesis: combined internal-external fixation. Foot Ankle Int 2001;22:92–7.
6. Adams JC. Arthrodesis of the ankle joint: experiences with transfibular approach. J Bone Joint Surg 1948;30(B):506–11.
7. Frankel JP, Bacardi BE. Chevron ankle arthrodesis with bone grafting and internal fixation. J Foot Surg 1986;25:234–40.
8. Anderson R. Concentric arthrodesis of the ankle joint: a transmalleolar approach. J Bone Joint Surg 1945;27:37–48.
9. Baciu CC. A simple technique for arthrodesis of the ankle. J Bone Joint Surg 1986;68(B):266–7.
10. Campbell P. Arthrodesis of the ankle with modified distraction-compression and bone-grafting. J Bone Joint Surg 1990;72:552–6.
11. Campbell CJ, Rinehart WT, Kalenak A. Arthrodesis of the ankle: deep autogenous inlay grafts with maximum cancellous bone apposition. J Bone Joint Surg 1974; 56:63–70.
12. Vogler HW. Ankle fusion: techniques and complications. J Foot Surg 1991; 30:80–4.

13. Thordarson DB, Markolf KL, Cracchiolo A. Arthrodesis of the ankle with cancellous-bone screws and fibular strut graft. Biomechanical analysis. J Bone Joint Surg 1990;72:1359–63.

14. Mauerer RC, Cimino WR, Cox CV, et al. Transarticular cross-screw fixation; a technique of ankle arthrodesis. Clin Orthop 1991;268:56–69.

15. Morgan CD, Henke JA, Bailey RW, et al. Long-term results of tibiotalar arthrodesis. J Bone Joint Surg 1985;67:546–50.

16. Mears DC, Gordon RG, Kann SE, et al. Ankle arthrodesis with an anterior tension plate. Clin Orthop 1991;268:70–7.

17. Paremain GD, Miller SD, Myerson MS. Ankle arthrodesis: results after the miniarthrotomy technique. Foot Ankle Int 1996;17:247–51.

18. Frey C, Halikus NM, Vu-Rose T, et al. A review of ankle arthrodesis: predisposing factors to nonunion. Foot Ankle Int 1994;15(11):581–4.

19. Morrey BF, Wiedeman GP Jr. Complications and long-term results of ankle arthrodeses following trauma. J Bone Joint Surg Am 1980;62(5):777–84.

20. O'Brien TS, Hart TS, Shereff MJ, et al. Open versus arthroscopic ankle arthrodesis: a comparative study. Foot Ankle Int 1999;20(6):368–74.

21. Stone JW. Arthroscopic ankle arthrodesis. Foot Ankle Clin 2006;11(2):361–8.

22. Collman DR, Kaas MH, Schuberth JM. Arthroscopic ankle arthrodesis: factors influencing union in 39 consecutive patients. Foot Ankle Int 2006;27:1079–85.

23. Winson IG, Robinson DE, Allen PE. Arthroscopic ankle arthrodesis. J Bone Joint Surg Br 2005;87(3):343–7.

24. Kats J, van Kampen A, de Waal-Malefijt MC. Improvement in technique for arthroscopic ankle fusion: results in 15 patients. Knee Surg Sports Traumatol Arthrosc 2003;11(1):46–9.

25. Dent CM, Patil M, Fairclough JA. Arthroscopic ankle arthrodesis. J Bone Joint Surg Br 1993;75(5):830–2.

26. Gougoulias NE, Agathangelidis FG, Parsons SW. Arthroscopic ankle arthrodesis. Foot Ankle Int 2007;28(6):695–706.

27. Ferkel RD, Hewitt M. Long-term results of arthroscopic ankle arthrodesis. Foot Ankle Int 2005;26(4):275–80.

28. Ogilvie-Harris DJ, Lieberman I, Fitsialos D. Arthroscopically assisted arthrodesis for osteoarthrotic ankles. J Bone Joint Surg Am 1993;75(8):1167–74.

29. Zvijac JE, Lemak L, Schurhoff MR, et al. Analysis of arthroscopically assisted ankle arthrodesis. Arthroscopy 2002;18(1):70–5.

30. Berk TA, van Baal MCPM, Sturkenboom JM, et al. Functional outcomes and quality of life in patients with post-traumatic arthrosis undergoing open or arthroscopic talocrural arthrodesis-a retrospective cohort with prospective follow-up. J Foot Ankle Surg 2022;61(3):609–14.

31. Morelli F, Princi G, Cantagalli MR, et al. Arthroscopic vs open ankle arthrodesis: a prospective case series with seven years follow-up. World J Orthop 2021;12(12):1016–25.

32. Schneider D. Arthroscopic ankle fusion. Arthroscopic Video J 1983;3.

33. Salk RS, Chang TJ, D'Costa WF, et al. Sodium hyaluronate in the treatment of osteoarthritis of the ankle: a controlled, randomized, double-blind pilot study. J Bone Joint Surg Am 2006;88(2):295–302.

34. Smith PA. Intra-articular autologous conditioned plasma injections provide safe and efficacious treatment for knee osteoarthritis: an FDA-sanctioned, randomized, double-blind, placebo-controlled clinical trial. Am J Sports Med 2016;44(4):884–91.

35. Paget LDA, Reurink G, de Vos R, et al. Effect of platelet-rich plasma injections vs placebo on ankle symptoms and function in patients with ankle osteoarthritis: a randomized clinical trial. JAMA 2021;326(16):1595–605.
36. Stetson WB, Ferkel RD. Ankle arthroscopy: II. Indications and results. J Am Acad Orthop Surg 1996;4(1):24–34.
37. Tang KL, Li QH, Chen GX, et al. Arthroscopically assisted ankle fusion in patients with end-stage tuberculosis. Arthroscopy 2007;23(9):919–22.
38. Issac RT, Thomson LE, Khan K, et al. Do degree of coronal plane deformity and patient related factors affect union and outcome of Arthroscopic versus Open Ankle Arthrodesis? Foot Ankle Surg 2022;28(5):635–41.
39. Schmid T, Krause F, Penner MJ, et al. Effect of preoperative deformity on arthroscopic and open ankle fusion outcomes. Foot Ankle Int 2017;38(12):1301–10.
40. Myerson MS, Quill G. Ankle arthrodesis. A comparison of an arthroscopic and an open method of treatment. Clin Orthop Relat Res 1991;268(268):84–95.
41. Mann RA, Van Manen JW, Wapner K, et al. Ankle fusion. Clin Orthop Relat Res 1991;268:49–55.
42. Glick JM, Morgan CD, Myerson MS, et al. Ankle arthrodesis using an arthroscopic method: long-term follow-up of 34 cases. Arthroscopy 1996;12(4):428–34.
43. Jay RM. A new concept of ankle arthrodesis via arthroscopic technique. Clin Podiatr Med Surg 2000;17(1):147–57.
44. Monroe MT, Beals TC, Manoli A 2nd. Clinical outcome of arthrodesis of the ankle using rigid internal fixation with cancellous screws. Foot Ankle Int 1999;20(4):227–31.
45. Crosby LA, Yee TC, Formanek TS, et al. Complications following arthroscopic ankle arthrodesis. Foot Ankle Int 1996;17:340–2.
46. Corso SJ, Zimmer TJ. Technique and clinical evaluation of arthroscopic ankle arthrodesis. Arthroscopy 1995;11:585–90.
47. Jerosch J, Steinbeck J, Schroder M, et al. Arthroscopically assisted arthrodesis of the ankle joint. Arch Orthop Trauma Surg 1996;115:182–9.
48. Brown CW, Orme TJ, Richardson HD. The rate of pseudoarthrosis (surgical nonunion) in patients who are smokers and patients who are nonsmokers; a comparison study. Spine 1986;11:942–3.
49. Glasman SD, Anagnost SC, Parker A, et al. The effect of cigarette smoking and smoking cessation on spinal fusion. Spine 2000;25:2608–15.
50. Haverstock BD, Mandracchia VJ. Cigarette smoking and bone healing: implication in foot and ankle surgery. J Foot Ankle Surg 1998;37:69–74.
51. Ishikawa SN, Murphy GA, Richardson EG. The effect of cigarette smoking on hindfoot fusions. Foot Ankle Int 2002;23:996–8.
52. Nolan J, Jenkins RA, Kurihara K, et al. The acute effects of cigareete smoke exposure on experimental skin flaps. Plast Reconst Surg 1985;75:544–51.
53. Sherwin MA, Gastwirth CM. Detrimental effects of cigarette smoking on lower extremity wound healing. J Foot Surg 1990;29:84–7.
54. Cobb TK, Gabrielsen TA, Campbell DC 2nd, et al. Cigarette smoking and nonunion after ankle arthrodesis. Foot Ankle 1994;15:64–7.
55. Jain SK, Tiernan D, Kearns SR. Analysis of risk factors for failure of arthroscopic ankle fusion in a series of 52 ankles. Foot Ankle Surg 2016;22(2):91–6.
56. DeVriese L, Dereymaeker G, Fabry G. Arthroscopic ankle arthrodesis preliminary report. Acta Orthop Belg 1994;60:389–92.
57. Blair HC. Comminuted fractures and fracture-dislocations of the body of the astragalus: operative treatment. Am J Surg 1943;59:37–43.

58. Honnenahalli Chandrappa M, Hajibandeh S, Hajibandeh S. Ankle arthrodesis-open versus arthroscopic: a systematic review and meta-analysis. J Clin Orthop Trauma 2017;8(Suppl 2):S71–7.
59. Turan I, Wredmark T, Fellander-Tsai L. Arthroscopic ankle arthrodesis in rheumatoid arthritis. Clin Orthop 1995;320:110–4.
60. Petersen KS, Lee MS, Buddecke DE. Arthroscopic versus open ankle arthrodesis: a retrospective cost analysis. J Foot Ankle Surg 2010;49:242–7.
61. Nielsen KK, Linde F, Jensen NC. The outcome of arthroscopic and open surgery ankle arthrodesis: a comparative retrospective study on 107 patients. Foot Ankle Surg 2008;14(3):153–7.
62. Townshend D, Di Silvestro M, Krause F, et al. Arthroscopic versus open ankle arthrodesis: a multicenter comparative case series. J Bone Joint Surg Am 2013;95(2):98–102.
63. Martinelli N, Bianchi A, Raggi G, et al. Open versus arthroscopic ankle arthrodesis in high-risk patients: a comparative study. Int Orthop 2022;46(3):515–21.
64. Veljkovic AN, Daniels TR, Glazebrook MA, et al. Outcomes of total ankle replacement, arthroscopic ankle arthrodesis, and open ankle arthrodesis for isolated non-deformed end-stage ankle arthritis. J Bone Joint Surg Am 2019;101(17):1523–9.

Posterior Arthroscopic Subtalar Joint Arthrodesis (Pasta)

Naohiro Shibuya, DPM, MS[a],*, Alden Simmons, DPM[b],
Frank Felix, DPM[b]

KEYWORDS

• Endoscopy • Arthroscopy • Fusion • Distraction • Push-pull

KEY POINTS

• Posterior arthroscopic subtalar joint arthrodesis (PASTA) can be used to minimize soft tissue trauma in vulnerable patient populations.

• PASTA preserves neurovascular structures of the sinus tarsi and tarsal canal, which can decrease nonunions, especially in high-risk patients including those who had a previous foot or ankle surgery in the proximity.

• PASTA preserves neurovascular structures of the sinus tarsi and tarsal canal, which can decrease the chance of future nonunions in the adjacent joints such as ankle and talonavicular joints.

• Although perception is that distraction of the subtalar joint is difficult, there are various techniques that allow for excellent exposure and access to the joint.

 Video content accompanies this article at http://www.podiatric.theclinics.com.

INTRODUCTION

Tasto was first to describe arthroscopic arthrodesis of the subtalar joint (STJ), and his technique utilized standard anterolateral and posterolateral portals.[1] In 2000, van Dijk and colleagues reported using posterior portals with the patient in a prone position.[2] Since then, many cases describing the posterior approach have been presented by different authors and surgeons. According to those case series, arthroscopic STJ arthrodesis results in good outcomes with a relatively low complication rate.[3–10] Fusion rates range from 84% to 99%.[10,11] Comparative analysis of open versus arthroscopic approaches demonstrate a significant decrease in time to fusion,

[a] University of Texas Rio Grande Valley, School of Podiatric Medicine; [b] Baylor Scott and White Memorial Hospital, Texas A&M Health Science Center
* Corresponding author.
E-mail address: naohiro.shibuya@utrgv.edu

Clin Podiatr Med Surg 40 (2023) 471–481
https://doi.org/10.1016/j.cpm.2023.02.002
0891-8422/23/© 2023 Elsevier Inc. All rights reserved.

decreased length of hospital stays, and faster return to activity.[12,13] This all provides a more manageable postoperative course in terms of recovery, healing, and activity.

Despite these benefits, the procedure is not common mostly due to the perception that the surgical procedure is difficult and time consuming. It may also result in more incomplete joint preparation compared with the open procedure.[14] Our aim is to describe the technique as well as to introduce tips and pearls that help surgeons to make this procedure more efficient and manageable in their practices. These tips help distract the joint at ease and provide workable space for the surgeon to prepare the joint for arthrodesis arthroscopically.

SURGICAL TECHNIQUE
Patient Positioning

With the PASTA procedure, as the name implies, the STJ is approached from the posterior side. Therefore, the patient is placed in a prone position. The feet are hanging off the end of the table to avoid hyperextension of the ankles. Although one may consider placing a bump under the anterior ankle to avoid the hyperextension without having the feet hanging off the table, this makes the access to the posterior facet of the STJ more difficult when the surgeon is positioned distal to the feet. Although protecting the bony anterior crests of the tibia during the procedure is important, a large cushion, such as a bulky pillow or blanket under the lower legs, makes the knee flexed and raises the lower leg. When the surgeon is positioned distal to the feet, arthroscopic instruments then need to be aimed toward the surgeon's body to align with the slope of the posterior facet of the STJ in order to get into the joint. This unnatural positioning of the instruments (normally, they are aimed away from the surgeon's body) can create an uncomfortable wrist position and body posture throughout the case. Use of a Wilson Frame can decline the lower legs and help with the surgeon's as well as the patient's comfort throughout the case. Alternatively, "lowering the feet" by placing the table in a more reverse-Trendelenburg position helps with the surgeon's posture. A sandbag or bump may be placed under the contralateral hip to internally rotate the operative lower extremity to position the foot straight up and down (**Fig. 1**).

A standard-sized c-arm fluoroscopy, rather than a mini-c-arm, is recommended. The c-arm can be placed to project the lateral view of the foot and left in that position throughout the duration of the procedure if desired (**Fig. 2**). With the larger c-arm, the

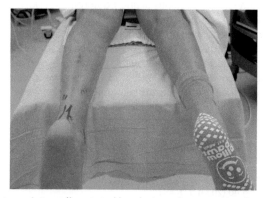

Fig. 1. The left foot was internally rotated by placing a bump under the contralateral hip to improve the access to the medial side of the posterior facet of the STJ.

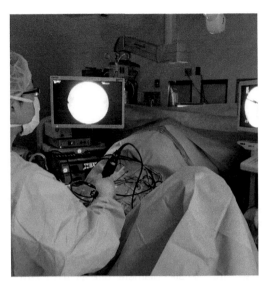

Fig. 2. The surgeon is positioned at the end of the table, a c-arm is positioned to take images of lateral views, and the monitors are positioned in front of the surgeon.

procedure does not have to be disrupted while c-arm images are taken. The surgeon does not have to put down the arthroscopic instruments while evaluating or taking c-arm images. The c-arm can be particularly useful to confirm the orientation of arthroscopic instruments; therefore, putting down the instruments while taking c-arm pictures is not desirable. Once becoming more comfortable and efficient with the PASTA technique, the need for the c-arm becomes negligible during positioning.

Initial Joint Exposure

Posterior-medial and posterior-lateral portals are then created just medial and lateral to the Achilles tendon (see **Fig. 2**). Unlike procedures such as the removal of os trigonum or treatment of posterior impingement syndrome, when access to the STJ is not needed arthroscopic instruments need to be aimed more plantarly to align with the orientation of the plantarly sloped STJ in PASTA. Therefore, the portals are placed approximately 1 to 2 cm proximal to the tip of the lateral malleolus and the instruments are slightly angulated plantarly to accommodate for the STJ orientation (**Fig. 3**). In a case of joint depressed, neglected calcaneal fracture, the portals are often lowered to accommodate for the lack of physiologic sloping of the posterior facet (**Fig. 4**). A spinal needle can be used to confirm the correct initial trajectory and portal placement by inserting the needle under live fluoroscopy into the STJ. This is particularly useful for posterior facets that are depressed.

Once portals are established, arthroscopic instruments are introduced. Unlike an ankle arthroscopic procedure, the STJ cannot be inflated with fluid to allow easy access to the joint by the instruments. Therefore, the joint is initially visualized from the outside, and the joint capsule as well as posterior ligaments are transected to access the STJ. In other words, the initial part of the procedure takes place outside the joint utilizing endoscopic techniques.

It is recommended to use a larger-bored lens, such as the one in a 4.0 mm by 30° arthroscope in this area. The large cannula over the lens also allows more inflow of fluid into the area outside of the joint to "push" the soft tissue (mainly subcutaneous

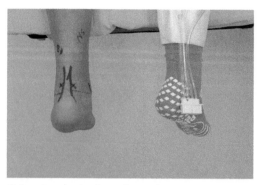

Fig. 3. Posterior-medial and posterior-lateral portals are positioned just medial and lateral to the Achilles tendon to avoid tibial vessels and the nerve medially and the sural nerve and small saphenous vein laterally.

adipose tissue) and permits more clear visualization in front of the lens. The 4.0-mm lens, when compared with a smaller diameter one as in a 2.7-mm scope, also allows greater field of view, which makes the procedure more efficient. The perception is that the larger-bore arthroscope is more difficult to be inserted in the STJ but there are many tips that allow this to be manageable.

Triangulation of instruments is now performed. Again, this will not take place in the joint; rather, an instrument is identified in the soft tissue posterior to the joint. An arthroscope can enter from either portal, and an instrument, such as a hemostat, can come in from the other portal. Aiming the instruments toward the second digit of the foot allows for good initial trajectory to the posterior aspect of the STJ. A hemostat can be utilized to spread the soft tissue and to puncture the intermuscular septum

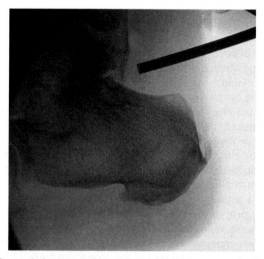

Fig. 4. The level of portal placement is crucial in posteriorly approached arthroscopic subtalar joint arthrodesis (PASTA) as the orientation of the instruments need to match with the angulation of the posterior facet of the STJ. In a typical foot with no history of trauma, the portals are placed approximately 1 to 2 cm proximal to the tip of the lateral malleolus and the instruments are slightly angulated plantarly.

and guide the arthroscope deeper into the area. Once the instrument is identified with triangulation, the image on the screen can be focused using the focus dial or autofocus button using the contrast between the soft tissue and the instrument. A shaver can then remove soft tissue in front of the arthroscope for visualization. Once the space is created in front of the lens, the arthroscope is advanced deeper into the created space. The process is repeated until it reaches the back of the STJ. Along with the 4.0 mm arthroscope, a larger-diameter shaver is recommended because it is less prone to clogging up the suctioning canal of the instrument with the soft tissue. It is also recommended that the shaver to have aggressive teeth because the sharp serrated edge of the shaver is more effective in cutting through the tough posterior ligamentous structures. If necessary, the instruments can follow the superior surface of the posterior tuberosity of the calcaneus for an orientation purpose to find the posterior aspect of the STJ.

If unfamiliar with the posterior ankle arthroscopy, the flexor hallucis longus tendon should be identified before the transection of the posterior ligamentous and capsular structures to access the STJ (Video 1). The vital neurovascular structures are located just medial to the tendon; therefore, the rest of the procedure is to be performed lateral to the tendon. It should be noted that some patients have the neurovascular bundle more laterally and superficially, therefore the location of the vital structures can vary slightly among patients. It is conceivable that patients with severe chronic pes planus deformity can have the neurovascular structures located more closer to the working portals. After the safe zone is established, the shaver or biter/basket grasper is utilized to debride the posterior ligamentous and capsular structures of the STJ.

Arthrofibrosis, pathologic stiffening of a joint caused by excessive inflammatory process, can be encountered at the posterior capsule in some patients. This happens particularly in patients who have a history of trauma or surgery in the proximity. A fibrosed capsule is a thick, cord-like structure spanning the talus and the calcaneus. Less matured fibrosis seems more like a scar. It can also be calcified and impenetrable by some of the instruments used for soft tissues. Osteotomes may be necessary to release and expose the posterior facet in that situation. Large, calcified segments are resected and removed in small pieces with a grasper or pituitary rongeur. In cases of a previous calcaneal fracture, osteophytosis, malunion of small fragments, or depressed STJ can make it difficult to access the joint. An arthroscopic osteotome and a mallet are utilized to remove the osseous portion that is blocking the access to the posterior facet of the STJ (Video 2).

Once the posterior aspect of the posterior facet of the STJ is clearly visualized, the joint is placed through its range of motion to confirm the joint is indeed the STJ. Due to the proximity of the ankle joint viewed from the posterior aspect, one can easily confuse it with the STJ.

Joint Distraction

Distraction of the STJ can be achieved using one of the following techniques.

Gravity distraction

Gravity distraction involves the patient in the prone position with the foot hanging off the edge of the bed, allowing gravity to distract the joint.[7] This technique can be used when there is an adequate joint space for the instrumentation to complete the synovectomy, debridement, and joint preparation. When there is not enough space, an external foot strap can be utilized for further distraction. Normally, this technique is not adequate for an average STJ to perform arthrodesis with the posterior approach.

Blunt trocar (shuck and hold) technique

A blunt trocar can be used to further distract the STJ.[15] The trocar is inserted from a separate portal and forced into the STJ to achieve separation of the talar and calcaneal surfaces of the posterior facet. A separate stub incision is made just posterior to the peroneal tendons but anterior to the sural nerve, approximately 2 to 3 cm from the tip of the lateral malleolus. A trocar is then inserted from the third incision and identified using the triangulation technique at the posterior aspect of the STJ. The trocar is then advanced into the posterior facet to "wedge-open" the joint (**Fig. 5**). As initial distraction is limited by the thickness of the trocar, a larger trocar is more advantageous. However, a small trocar may be necessary initially to "loosen" the joint before insertion of the larger one. A blunt trocar is preferable for deeper insertion into the joint without catching the cartilage or subchondral bone with the sharp tip along the way. Once the trocar is inserted deeply in the posterior facet, it can be used as a lever to temporarily ply-open the joint (with the similar maneuver as shucking an oyster). The temporarily distracted joint can be then held in place with a Steinmann pin spanning across the joint (Video 3).

Skeletal traction

Another option is calcaneal skeletal traction. A transfixation wire is placed in the calcaneal tuberosity. The wire is pulled through a traction device to distract the STJ. Different modifications of the technique have been described[16–18]; however, the joint capsule and interosseous ligaments need to be released circumferentially to achieve good distraction using this technique. It should also be noted that the traction force is dissipated by distraction of ankle joint first, often losing effectiveness.

"Push-pull" distraction technique

The push-pull technique, described by Shibuya and colleagues, utilizes a fully threaded cortical screw to push the talus while the calcaneus is pulled proximally to distract the joint.[19] In authors' opinion, this technique gives the easiest and most effective distraction of the STJ in preparation for arthrodesis.

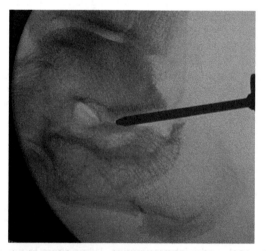

Fig. 5. In a neglected calcaneal fracture, the joint is often depressed (and the arthritic posterior facet is more parallel to the ground); therefore, the portals are often lowered to adjust for the lack of physiologic sloping.

This too requires a third stab incision created at the retro-lateral malleolar area, just posterior to the peroneal tendons, to perform a "predistraction" using the blunt trocar technique descried above.[15] From this portal, a trocar is again inserted and advanced toward the posterior lateral aspect of the posterior facet of the STJ. The trocar is then identified under arthroscopy and inserted into the posterior facet (Video 4). This will in turn distract the joint to some degree (see **Fig. 4**). This "predistraction" allows visualization of the STJ while performing the next step, insertion of a "push-pull" screw.

After the "predistraction," the calcaneal tuberosity is under-drilled with an appropriate-sized drill for the screw being utilized. It is drilled from the plantar-posterior aspect of the calcaneal tuberosity, through a stab incision, toward the posterior facet of the STJ (as if a screw is inserted to fixate the STJ). Although many types of screws work to for this technique, it should be noted that the screw must be long enough to reach and distract the STJ and its thread length needs to be longer than the amount of desired distraction. A non–self-tapping solid screw is preferable but not required. Typically, a 70 to 80-mm screw, either fully threaded or long-threaded (>20 mm) with greater than 4.0 mm diameter, is used. A self-tapping/self-drilling screw may unwantedly penetrate into the talus before significant amount of distraction can be achieved, and a cannulated screw causes water leak through the hollow shaft.

Under-drilling is performed only in the calcaneus (**Fig. 6**). The drill hole is oriented as if a screw is inserted for a subtalar fusion in the posterior facet from the posterior-plantar to dorsal-anterior orientation. More effective distraction can be achieved if the screw is oriented perpendicular to the posterior facet.

Next, the screw is inserted through the drill hole from the plantar-posterior aspect of the calcaneus. Once the screw is advanced to the STJ, the tip of the screw is visualized under arthroscopy. The screw is slowly advanced until it hits the talar surface of the posterior facet. As the screw is advanced further, it pushes the talus away from the calcaneus. Because the screw does not advance into the talus due to lack of a drill hole in the talus, it distracts the joint (Video 5). The screw therefore "pushes" the talus while it "pulls" the calcaneus away. Once desired distraction is achieved, the advancement is discontinued (**Fig. 7**). For more powerful distraction, the push-pull

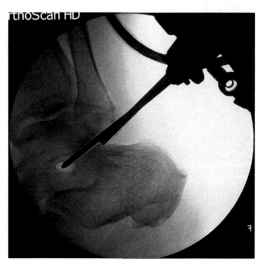

Fig. 6. Wedge-opening the STJ via a trocar.

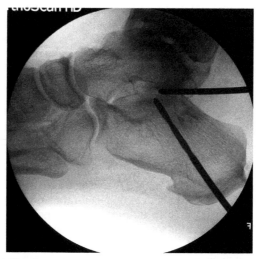

Fig. 7. The under-drill is through the calcaneus, reaching the STJ but not penetrating into the talus.

screw can be placed more posteriorly; however, if planning to utilize this push-pull screw as a second point of fixation at the end of the procedure, it is recommended to place the under-drill exactly where the second point of fixation is desired. If the screw is placed more anteriorly in the posterior facet, the distraction power is weaker; however, it gives more space to work with the arthroscopic instruments in the joint.

When using a self-tapping/drilling screw, the tip of the screw may unintentionally self-drill into the talus on contact when the STJ is extremely tight. To avoid this, the trocar, which was used for the initial "predistraction," may be utilized as a joystick to further "predistract" the joint while advancing the screw. With this predistracting method, the screw acts as a "stopper" to maintain the distraction as in the "shuck and hold" technique (**Fig. 8**).

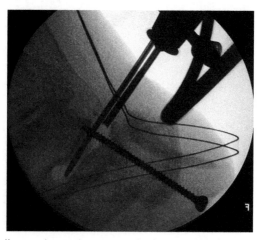

Fig. 8. The push-pull screw is creating a space in the posterior facet of the STJ.

Joint Preparation and Fixation

Although the joint is distracted, the joint is prepared for arthrodesis. Typically, only the posterior facet is prepared while the middle and anterior facets are not prepared. When arthrodesis is needed for nonarthritic joints, there is a significant amount of cartilage that needs to be removed. Both curved and straight arthroscopic osteotomes are useful to peel off a large portion of the cartilage effectively. Once getting closer to the sinus tarsi area, an angle curette can be used to remove the cartilage by pulling the instrument from anterior to posterior so that the cartilage is not pushed into the sinus tarsi. It is important not to violate the content in the neurovascular-rich sinus tarsi space. Once the cartilage is removed, the subchondral bone is violated to achieve bleeding surfaces. An unhooded bur of 3.0 mm to 4.0 mm is recommended, as these tend to reach different areas of the STJ more easily. The hood of the bur oftentimes gets in a way and does not allow deep penetration past the subchondral plate in some areas of the STJ depending on the angle. The bur can be used to create golf-ball-like dimples by burying the tip of the bur down into the cancellous bone underneath the subchondral plate. A curved osteotome may be used to "fish-scale" some hard-to-reach places. In an arthritic STJ, where there is no significant amount of cartilage left, a bur can be used right away to denude the remaining cartilage and subchondral bone at the same time. After the joint is prepped, the joint is inspected to make sure the whole posterior facet is exposed to bleeding cancellous bone.

Authors often use osteoconductive bone substitute in the STJ to fill those golf-ball-like dimples. The material needs to be flowable into the joint space so that it can be delivered through a small cannula that fits through one of the portals. The process can be visualized via an arthroscope inserted from the other portal (Video 6) or through fluoroscopy when a radio-opaque material is used. Once the osteoconductive material is injected in the joint space, the STJ is fixated. If the "push-pull" screw was used, the screw can be removed at this point. If desired, the screw can be advanced into the talus as a second point of fixation after a primary fixation is placed elsewhere. When a self-tapping/drilling screw is utilized for the push-pull technique, the screw can be backed out until the joint is undistracted and a separate primary compression screw is inserted across the joint elsewhere using the standard fixation technique. Once stable fixation is achieved from the primary fixation, the "push-pull" screw is advanced into the talus as a second point of fixation. If it starts to distract the joint despite the primary fixation, the screw needs to be removed completely and the under-drill needs to be completed in the talus, before reinsertion of the screw. If a non–self-tapping/drilling screw was used for the push-pull technique, it too needs to be removed completely and the talus is under-drilled before the reinsertion of the screw.

SUMMARY

During an open procedure, a surgeon may sacrifice collateral, posterior, and interosseous ligaments to adequately distract the STJ. Over releasing of these structures may violate the vasculature in the sinus tarsi and canalis tarsi. Posterior arthroscopic STJ arthrodesis preserves the major vascular supply to the talus by avoiding the deltoid branch and arteries to sinus tarsi and tarsal canal.

A disadvantage of using the posterior arthroscopic approach is that joint distraction can be difficult with the traditional techniques. An ankle distractor does not easily overcome the tightness of the STJ. The distraction force is dispersed mainly in the ankle joint before the STJ can be distracted. The trocar technique is a useful distraction method that works in most cases,[15] but frequent loosening/slippage of the trocar and inadequate distraction of the medial side can be a problem in stiffer STJs. Therefore, the "shuck-and-hold" or "push-pull" screw technique can be utilized to provide stable and powerful distraction without slippage or extensive release of capsular or ligamentous structures. The screw can also be converted to a second point of fixation after the primary compression screw is placed.

Although most primary arthrodesis techniques of the STJ have a high union rate, a well vascularized talus and noncompromised skin is crucial if future procedures, such as adjacent joint arthrodesis (namely talonavicular and tibiotalar joints) or total ankle arthroplasty, are needed. If a surgeon suspects a need of future procedures, he/she can consider this approach. Historically, arthroscopy of STJ is not a common procedure due to the perception of difficulty in distraction. However, with use of these special techniques, one can find this procedure much more manageable.

CLINICS CARE POINTS

- Initial positioning of patient is crucial for successful joint access.
- A larger size of arthroscope allows for improved visualization of the joint and posterior capsule.
- If a patient has history of trauma, arthrofibrosis of the posterior STJ capsule can be expected. This makes the exposure of the posterior facet difficult technically.
- The length of the push-pull screw should be about the length of the normal STJ fixation screw.
- Distraction will be more powerful if push-pull screw is aimed more posteriorly in the posterior facet while more anterior position can allow a larger space to work arthroscopically.
- Combination of "shuck and hold" and "push-pull" technique gives the maximum distraction.
- The push-pull screw can be reinserted as a secondary point of fixation at the end of the procedure.

DISCLOSURE

None.

SUPPLEMENTARY DATA

Supplementary data related to this article can be found online at https://doi.org/10.1016/j.cpm.2023.02.002.

REFERENCES

1. Tasto JP, Frey C, Laimans P, et al. Arthroscopic ankle arthrodesis. Instr Course Lect 2000;49:259–80.
2. van Dijk CN, Scholten PE, Krips R. A 2-portal endoscopic approach for diagnosis and treatment of posterior ankle pathology. Arthroscopy 2000;16(8):871–6.
3. Ahn JH, Lee SK, Kim KJ, et al. Subtalar arthroscopic procedures for the treatment of subtalar pathologic conditions: 115 consecutive cases. Orthopedics 2009; 32(12):891.
4. Albert A, Deleu PA, Leemrijse T, et al. Posterior arthroscopic subtalar arthrodesis: ten cases at one-year follow-up. Orthop Traumatol Surg Res 2011;97(4):401–5.

5. El Shazly O, Nassar W, El Badrawy A. Arthroscopic subtalar fusion for post-traumatic subtalar arthritis. Arthroscopy 2009;25(7):783–7.

6. Frey C, Feder KS, DiGiovanni C. Arthroscopic evaluation of the subtalar joint: does sinus tarsi syndrome exist? Foot Ankle Int 1999;20(3):185–91.

7. Lee KB, Park CH, Seon JK, et al. Arthroscopic subtalar arthrodesis using a posterior 2-portal approach in the prone position. Arthroscopy 2010;26(2):230–8.

8. Lundeen RO. Arthroscopic fusion of the ankle and subtalar joint. Clin Podiatr Med Surg 1994;11(3):395–406.

9. Muraro GM, Carvajal PF. Arthroscopic arthodesis of subtalar joint. Foot Ankle Clin 2011;16(1):83–90.

10. Banerjee S, Gupta A, Elhence A, et al. Arthroscopic subtalar arthrodesis as a treatment strategy for subtalar arthritis: a systematic review. J Foot Ankle Surg 2021;60(5):1023–8.

11. Walter RP, Walker RW, Butler M, et al. Arthroscopic subtalar arthrodesis through the sinus tarsi portal approach: a series of 77 cases. Foot Ankle Surg 2018;24(5): 417–22.

12. Rungprai C, Phisitkul P, Femino JE, et al. Outcomes and complications after open versus posterior arthroscopic subtalar arthrodesis in 121 patients. J Bone Joint Surg Am 2016;98(8):636–46.

13. Rungprai C, Jaroenarpornwatana A, Chaiprom N, et al. Outcomes and complications of open vs posterior arthroscopic subtalar arthrodesis: a prospective randomized controlled multicenter study. Foot Ankle Int 2021;42(11):1371–83.

14. Chinnakkannu K, McKissack H, Alexander B, et al. Subtalar joint preparation using the Two Portal posterior arthroscopic technique versus the sinus tarsi Open approach: a cadaver study. Foot 2021;46:101690.

15. Lee KB, Saltzman CL, Suh JS, et al. A posterior 3-portal arthroscopic approach for isolated subtalar arthrodesis. Arthroscopy 2008;24(11):1306–10.

16. Beals TC, Junko JT, Amendola A, et al. Minimally invasive distraction technique for prone posterior ankle and subtalar arthroscopy. Foot Ankle Int 2010;31(4): 316–9.

17. Kim HN, Ryu SR, Park JM, et al. Subtalar arthroscopy with calcaneal skeletal traction in a hanging position. J Foot Ankle Surg 2012;51(6):816–9.

18. Rubin LG. Subtalar joint arthroscopy. Clin Podiatr Med Surg 2011;28(3):539–50.

19. Shibuya N, Smith RS, Escobedo LA, et al. A push-pull distraction method for arthroscopic subtalar joint arthrodesis. J Foot Ankle Surg 2014;53(6):825–8.

Arthroscopic Cartilage Transplantation

Tyler Tewilliager, DPM, AACFAS*, Kevin Nguyen, DPM, AACFAS, Alan Ng, DPM, FACFAS

KEYWORDS

- Arthroscopy • Cartilage repair • Cartilage grafting • Osteochondral defect • OLT

KEY POINTS

- The majority of primary osteochondral lesions can be effectively treated arthroscopically.
- Cartilage grafting has shown promise in early stages of research; however, there are still limited data on the different products available.
- Numerous products and techniques are available for the treatment of osteochondral lesions of the talus—each with their own benefits and indications. Multiple off the shelf chondral allografts exist for the treatment of smaller lesions. There is unfortunately no accepted consensus on whether one is superior to another.

INTRODUCTION/BACKGROUND

Osteochondral lesions of the talus (OLTs) are typically the result of traumatic injury to the ankle joint because primary osteoarthritis (OA) of the ankle only accounts for approximately 7% to 9% of ankle OA.[1] Hyaline cartilage has an inherently poor regenerative capacity, the ankle in addition to this has cartilage that is thinner than that of the hips/knees. There are multiple theories as to why ankle cartilage is less susceptible to primary OA than hips or knees, one of which being that ankle cartilage has increased stiffness and decreased permeability due to increased proteoglycans and water, this provides increased resistance to mechanical load.[2] Because of the lack of regenerative capacity of hyaline cartilage, there has been a large focus on cartilage regeneration techniques, these techniques include but are not limited to bone marrow stimulation, cartilage auto/allografting, and cartilage transplantation via OATs or en bloc replacement. Oftentimes, if these aforementioned options fail or OA is too far advanced, then patients may require ankle arthrodesis or arthroplasty for more definitive treatment.

Cartilage itself is aneural, and often times the pain that comes from OLTs is related to inflammatory markers from the synovium and subchondral bone failure.[3] As we learn more about the nature of OLTs of the talus, assessing subchondral bone health

Advanced Orthopedics and Sports Medicine Specialists, 8101 East Lowry Boulevard Suite 230, Denver, CO 80230, USA
* Corresponding author.
E-mail address: ttewilliagerDPM@gmail.com

Clin Podiatr Med Surg 40 (2023) 483–494
https://doi.org/10.1016/j.cpm.2023.02.006
0891-8422/23/© 2023 Elsevier Inc. All rights reserved.
podiatric.theclinics.com

becomes an important factor in pain relief and longevity of repair. Arthroscopic examination and debridement with microfracture has long been considered the gold standard for first-line treatment. However, there are increasing concerns on the long-term impact on subchondral bone health of the talus after this procedure. The scope of this article will focus further on cartilage regenerative options outside of bone marrow stimulation techniques. Some of these newer techniques include autograft chondrocyte implantation (matrix-induced autologous chondrocyte implantation [MACI]/autologous chondrocyte implantation [ACI]), as well as, a number of allograft options such as particulated juvenile allograft cartilage (PJAC)–DeNovo NT (Zimmer-Biomet, Warsaw, IN, USA), cartilage matrices such as BioCartilage (Arthrex, Naples, FL, USA), and cryopreserved chondrocyte discs—ProChondrix (Stryker, Kalamazoo, MI, USA). The goal of these techniques/products is to resurface and assist with chondral regeneration and attempt to provide a long-term relief from these challenging lesions.

The challenges with developing new products and regenerative tissues for cartilage defects stems from the lack of self-healing of hyaline cartilage. Many newer products in development are now focusing on engineered scaffolds of different materials to attempt to stimulate native articular cartilage formation via bioreactors. Although we do have some scaffolds available commercially, continued research to improve these is still being performed.[4]

PERTINENT ANATOMY

The ankle joint functions as a hinge and is composed of 3 bones—the tibia, fibula, and talus.[5] These bones interface and articulate in a more congruent fashion than that of the knee.[6] In terms of cartilage characteristics, the ankle differs from the knee in that the cartilage thickness is more uniform and also thinner. Hyaline cartilage of the ankle joint has a mean thickness between 1 and 1.7 mm, whereas the knee ranges from 1.6 to 6 mm.[7,8] Due to these characteristics, this unfortunately lends the ankle joint at a higher likelihood of osteochondral injury and subsequent arthritis. Microfracturing is not a new or emerging procedure but remains a treatment option because it is inexpensive and requires little proficiency. It is largely accepted that it does, however, produces inferior fibrocartilage that has limited long-term benefit.[9,10]

The goal in the repair of OLTs is to return the patient to a pain-free state where they can continue to perform their activities of daily living. This, however, is a more difficult task because there is a paucity in the cause of pain related to OLTs. Van Dijk and colleagues suggest that pain related to OLTs is due to a hydrostatic pressure in the ankle. Because the tibia bears weight onto the talus, the OLT allows for fluid to enter into the underlying subchondral bone, causing pressure and cyst formation.[11] In this section, we will explore different techniques utilized at the author's institution for the arthroscopic treatment of OLTs.

PARTICULATED JUVENILE ALLOGRAFT CARTILAGE (DeNovo)

PJAC, (DeNovo NT), is a form of cartilage resurfacing technique to help restore a more normal cartilage in the treatment of OLTs and was introduced in 2007. PJAC is taken from donors who are aged younger than 13 years; due to the age of the donors, there is an increased chondrocyte density and can be up to 100 times more active than adult donor cells. PJAC is an off-the shelf allograft that has a shelf life of 49 days from procurement to expiration, there is enough allograft present in one package to fill approximately a 2.5 cm^2 osteochondral defect.[12–14] PJAC has been described for use in cartilage defects of the knee, talus, shoulder, hip as well as metatarsal-phalangeal joint. However, this section will focus primarily on OLTs. Both open and arthroscopic techniques have been described in the use of PJAC. The technique chosen depends on the location of the lesion, size of lesion, and comfort of the surgeon with each technique.[15] Ryan and colleagues[16] did a comparative study on open versus arthroscopic implantation of PJAC and found no significant difference at 2-year follow-up between the 2 groups, and both groups demonstrated improvement from baseline. At the author's institution, an arthroscopic technique is preferred because it requires smaller skin incisions and thus minimizes the chance of skin complications.

The author's arthroscopic approach is as detailed below: The patient is placed in a supine position on the operating room table with a hip bump as necessary to allow the ankle to sit in a neutral position. The procedure is performed under general or spinal anesthesia with a thigh tourniquet at 275 to 300 mm Hg, the patient is placed in a thigh holder and then prepped and draped in usual sterile fashion. A noninvasive ankle distractor is applied to the operative ankle, 10cc of lidocaine with epinephrine is injected into the ankle and standard anteromedial and anterolateral portals are performed. Ankle joint is debrided as needed, the OLT is then identified and debrided to subchondral bone and healthy margins. An abdominal CO_2 insufflator is used to assist in drying out the ankle joint; after drying the ankle, CO_2 flow is turned off, the OLT base is prepped with a thin layer of fibrin glue, the PJAC is then delivered via a 10-gauge cannula to the OLT and smoothed in a single layer with a freer elevator. After PJAC is in place an additional layer of fibrin glue is applied over the graft, CO_2 flow is turned back on and the fibrin glue is allowed to dry in its entirety. The site is then confirmed to be dry before the removal of operative limb from distraction and closure of arthroscopic portals. **Figs. 1–10** demonstrate this technique performed arthroscopically.

Although PJAC has been on the market for several years, there is still a lack of large-scale comparative studies. A 2017 MRI analysis of PJAC in the patella found 75% of

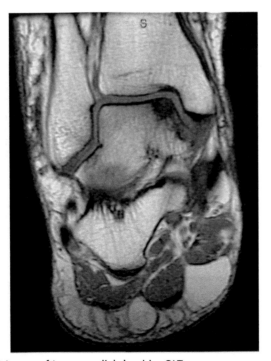

Fig. 1. Coronal T1 image of Large medial shoulder OLT.

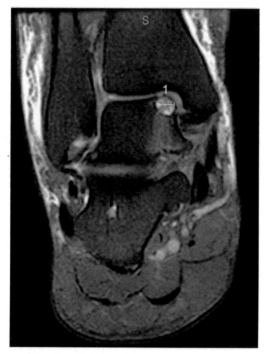

Fig. 2. Coronal T2 Imaging of medial shoulder OLT.

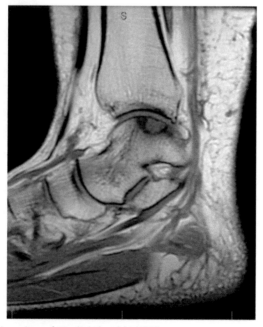

Fig. 3. Sagittal T1 imaging of Medial shoulder OLT.

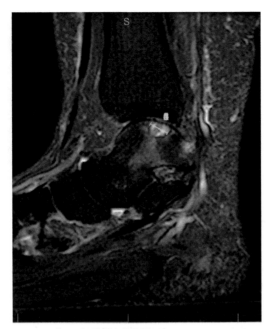

Fig. 4. Sagittal T2 imaging of medial shoulder OLT.

patients at 2-year follow-up had good-to-moderate filling of the defects with continued maturation of the graft during that time.[17] Multiple other smaller retrospective studies have shown good outcomes in the short term; however, the lack of significant long-term follow-up still remains. There are yet to be any comparative studies of PJAC versus adult autologous chips in a human population, 2 studies in animal models found no significant differences in the composition of the cartilage tissue at 6 months.[3]

DEHYDRATED ALLOGRAFT CARTILAGE SCAFFOLD (BioCartilage)

BioCartilage (Arthrex Inc, Naples, Florida) is another chondral allograft readily available in the form of dehydrated chips. This product offers a micronized cartilage

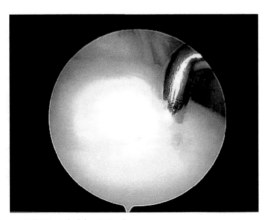

Fig. 5. Identification of OLT with blunt Probe.

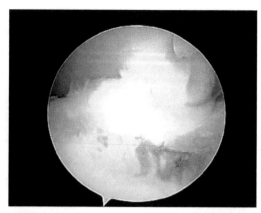

Fig. 6. Debridemtn of OLT to clean margins and bleeding subchondral bone.

matrix (MCM) with proteoglycans and type II collagen, which provides a bioactive scaffold for the formation of hyaline-like tissue.[18] BioCartilage is aseptically processed through a proprietary dehydration process that allows for storage at ambient temperatures with a shelf life of 5 years. Similar to other chondral allografts, BioCartilage may be delivered arthroscopically with the use of bone marrow aspirate concentrate (BMAC) or platelet rich plasma (PRP) to help encourage the differentiation of the cells into chondrocytes. As a micronized product, this graft is much finer than a particulated graft such as PJAC. As with PJACs, the OLTs are arthroscopically debrided in standard fashion and the BioCartilage is adhered to the site with fibrin glue.

In 2020, Shieh and colleagues studied the effects of MCM on cartilage repair with an in vitro study. After 3 weeks of culture, they observed that MCM mixed with mesenchymal stem cells (MSC) resulted in differentiated chondrocytes with more than 98% cell viability.[19] A retrospective study comparing the short-term outcomes of MCM + PRP/BMAC with that of isolated microfracture showed that augmenting microfracturing with MCM + PRP/BMAC significantly improved VAS and postoperative functional scores at a mean 4-year follow-up.[20]

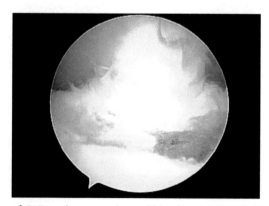

Fig. 7. Debridemtn of OLT to clean margins and bleeding subchondral bone.

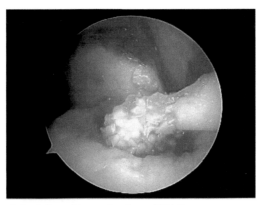

Fig. 8. Insufflation of the joint with application of PJAC.

CRYOPRESERVED OSTEOCHONDRAL ALLOGRAFT (ProChondrix)

ProChondrix (Stryker, Kalamazoo, MI, USA) is a minimally manipulated cryopreserved osteochondral allograft available in the form of precut discs, which contain viable chondrocytes, matrix, and growth factors. The product has a 2-year shelf life and comes in varying diameters from 11 mm to 20 mm.[21] ProChondrix may also be utilized and delivered to a lesion arthroscopically as well.

In 2019, Beth and colleagues reported on the application of ProChondrix in a 34-year-old woman with a 6.0 × 8.0 mm medial talar dome chondral lesion. At 12 months, repeat radiographs displayed complete resolution of the OTL, and the patient was back to performing preoperative activities without discomfort or disability.[22] Although promising in the short term, there is currently a paucity of literature on the product and further investigation is needed to determine effectiveness in the long term.

MATRIX-INDUCED AUTOLOGOUS CHONDROCYTE IMPLANTATION/AUTOLOGOUS CHONDROCYTE IMPLANTATION

ACI and the newer MACI are 2 techniques that involve harvesting autologous chondral tissue, culturing the cells, and then reimplanting them to fill chondral defects. These procedures are generally reserved for lesions larger than 1.5 cm^2 and innately require

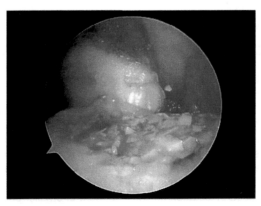

Fig. 9. Smoothing of PJAC into the OLT.

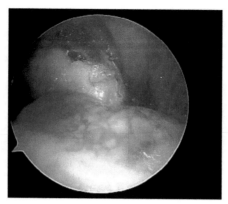

Fig. 10. Final seal of PJAC with Fibrin glue.

2 operations.[18] MACI has generally replaced ACI since matrix integration with the chondrocyte culture provides the required scaffold for cartilage growth, negating the need for a periosteal flap.[23]

The 2 procedures are similar in that the first stage involves acquiring a chondral sample arthroscopically, which is then sent for culture of the chondrocytes. The culturing process typically takes 3 to 4 weeks. The second stage is where the procedures differ. In ACI, an open procedure is usually required with a tibial or fibular osteotomy for reimplantation of the cultured chondrocytes. A periosteal flap is also required to create a bilayer in which the chondrocytes are applied and secured to the defect with fibrin glue.[24] MACI provides the advantage of nullifying the need for a periosteal flap or secondary scaffold. This is because during the culture stage, the new chondrocytes are grown on a matrix of type 1 and 3 collagen. The graft can then be secured with fibrin glue.[25]

In 2022, Yontar and colleagues published on the outcomes of MACI on 77 patients with a mean follow-up of 36 months. They concluded that in primary cases, there was a 95% success rate with high patient satisfaction. In revision cases, however, there was only a 61% success rate.[23] MACI and ACI provide the advantage of autogenous chondrocytes, which is thought to integrate and develop better. It unfortunately requires 2 separate procedures, which increases costs as well as the risks of surgery.

BONE MARROW ASPIRATE CONCENTRATE

Bone marrow aspirate concentrate (BMAC) is similar to PRP in that it is acquired from the host and is concentrated by centrifugation. However, BMAC has an advantage over PRP in that it contains MSCs, which have been shown to aid in the regeneration and growth of cartilage.[24] Similar to PRP, BMAC also contains platelets and thus provides a significant amount of growth factors such as PDGF and TGF-B. Both growth factors have been shown to aid in the growth and maturation of chondrocytes.[24,25] In an equine model, BMAC has been shown to provide full-thickness cartilage repair in extensive deficits (15-mm diameter lesions) when compared with microfracturing alone. The regenerated cartilage was not only better incorporated into the surrounding cartilage but was also thicker and smoother.[26]

BMAC may be used in isolation for the treatment of smaller chondral lesions or as an adjuvant to aid in hydration of allografts. When used as an adjuvant, BMAC can be used to rehydrate and coat the graft, providing a rich source of MSCs, which may help with graft incorporation and reduction of postoperative cyst formation.[27] In 2016, Chahla and colleagues published a systematic review on the outcomes of BMAC in the treatment of talar chondral lesions. Their review included 184 patients with a mean age of 29.5 years and an average follow-up of 34.3 months. The reviewed studies revealed that the use of BMAC as an adjunct in treatment of moderately sized OCLs was beneficial with no major complications.[25] In 2020, Vannini and colleagues published on the use of BMAC with a scaffold for the treatment of OLTs. At 10-year follow-up, they reported statistically significant improvements in AOFAS scores (mean 52.3–73.5). The authors concluded that this 1-step technique of articular debridement with implantation of a BMAC loaded scaffold provides a long-term improvement in patient reported outcomes.[28] Whether BMAC is used as an adjunct or in isolation, it provides a rich source of MSCs with a low complication rate and donor site morbidity. HYAFF-11 is a hyaluronic acid (HA)-based biomaterial that serves as a scaffold to fill chondral defects. Grigolo and colleagues evaluated the growth of chondrocytes on the HA scaffold at various intervals from 1 hour to 60 days. The scaffolds were seeded with human articular knee cartilage and at 4 days, the entire scaffold surface was covered with chondrocytes. Utilizing immunochemistry and ultrastructural analysis, the authors found that the chondrocytes expressed and produced type 2 collagen and aggrecan, as well as a downregulation of type 1 collagen.[29] In 2017, Sadlik and colleagues followed up on the utilization of HA as a BMAC carrier in a 1-step technique for OLT repairs. The authors performed the procedure arthroscopically in the repair of chondral lesions with underlying subchondral bone loss. The bone defects were debrided and filled with autologous graft. The articular cartilage was then repaired with an HA embedded BMAC graft. Although the technique was performed in knees, the authors state that the procedure has been successful for lesions 3 to 4 cm^2, which may also prove to be a viable option in treatment of talar OCLs. At 5-year follow-up, there were significant improvements in outcome scores with maintained scores at final follow-up when compared with microfracture alone.[30,31] There are several HA products, such as Hyalofast (Anika, Bedford, MA) that are currently being utilized around the world. In the United States, there are clinical trials being conducted which will hopefully provide additional options in the future.

SUMMARY

Treatment of OLTs remains a hot topic of debate, whereas many newer ideas lean away from treatment of these with microfracture due to long-term subchondral bone failure this is still considered by many to be the gold-standard first-stage treatment. When bone marrow stimulation techniques alone have failed, there are several grafting options available; however, there is no definitive best product on the market for the treatment of these. MACI/ACI focuses on utilizing the patient's own cartilage as graft but requires multiple operations to be performed. Multiple allograft options are available on the market including but not limited to the ones discussed above; the biggest challenge with these are the lack of long-term comparative studies. Some of the newer treatment options for cartilage restoration are in the form of engineered scaffolds; however, there is still significant development of these being performed and the perfect material for cartilage growth has yet to be reported. Although many grafting options are available, these lesions still present a significant challenge for both patient and surgeon and oftentimes require multiple operations during the course of the patient's lifetime.

CLINICS CARE POINTS

- A thorough history is necessary and helpful in making a diagnosis of OLTs. Clinical examinations positive for ankle "clicking" or "catching" should raise suspicion of chondral injury and defects.

- MRI is necessary for the evaluation of chondral lesions as well as the stability of the underlying subchondral bone.

- In the author's institution, microfracturing is avoided because it destabilized the subchondral bone and may lead to cystic formations. If there is concern for subchondral instability, subchondroplasty is performed.

- Abrasion chondroplasty with the detailed techniques mentioned are the mainstay treatments for OLTs.

- Patients are typically weight-bearing at 2 weeks. High impact is avoided until 4 months postop because the chondral allografts are still incorporating.

DISCLOSURE

A. Ng is a paid consultant of Zimmer Biomet.

REFERENCES

1. Valderrabano V, Horisberger M, Russell I, et al. Etiology of ankle arthritis. Clin Orthop Relat Res 2009;467(7):1800–6.
2. Anderson DD, Chubinskaya S, Guilak F, et al. Post-traumatic osteoarthritis:improved understanding and opportunities for early intervention. J Orthop Res 2011;29(6):802–9.
3. Christensen B, Olesen M, et al. Particulated cartilage for chondral and osteochondral repair: a review. Cartilage 2021;13(1):1047–57.
4. Wei W, Dai H. Articular cartilage and osteochondral tissue engineering techniques: recent advances and challenges. Bioact Mater 2021;6:4830–55.
5. Kraeutler MJ, Kaenkumchorn T, Pascual-Garrido C, et al. Peculiarities in ankle cartilage. Cartilage 2017;8(1):12–8.
6. Hendren L, Beeson P. A review of the differences between normal and osteoarthritis articular cartilage in human knee and ankle joints. Foot 2009;19(3):171–6.
7. Shepherd DE, Seedhom BB. Thickness of human articular cartilage in joints of the lower limb. Ann Rheum Dis 1999 Jan;58(1):27–34.
8. Millington SA, Grabner M, Wozelka R, et al. Quantification of ankle articular cartilage topography and thickness using a high resolution stereophotography system. Osteoarthr Cartil 2007;15(2):205–11.
9. Yanke AB, Chubinskaya S. The state of cartilage regeneration: current and future technologies. Curr Rev Musculoskelet Med 2015;8(1):1–8.
10. Goyal D, Keyhani S, Lee EH, et al. Evidence-based status of microfracture technique: a systematic review of level I and II studies. Arthroscopy 2013;29(9):1579–88.
11. van Dijk CN, Reilingh ML, Zengerink M, et al. Osteochondral defects in the ankle: why painful? Knee Surg Sports Traumatol Arthrosc 2010;18(5):570–80.
12. Ng A, Bernherd K. The use of particulated juvenile allograft cartilage in foot and ankle surgery. Clin Podiatr Med Surg 2018;35:11–8.
13. Aldawsari K, Alrabai H, et al. Role of particulated juvenile cartilage allograft transplantaion in osteochondral lesions of the talus: a systematic review. Foot Ankle Surg 2021;27:10–4.

14. Adkisson H, Martin J, Amendola R, et al. The potential of human allogenic juvenile chondrocytes for restoration of articular cartilage. Am J Sports Med 2010;38(7): 1324–33.

15. Adams S, Easley M, Schon L. Particulated juvenile articular cartilage allograft transplantation for osteochondral lesions of the talus. Oper Tech Orthop 2014; 24(3):181–9.

16. Ryan P, Turner R, et al. Comparative outcomes for the treatment of articular cartilage lesions in the ankle with a DeNovo NT natural tissue graft. The Orthopedic Journal of Sports Medicine 2018;6(12):1–6.

17. Grawe B, Burge A, et al. Cartilage regeneration in full-thickness patellar chondral defects treated with particulated juvenile articular allograft cartilage: an MRI analysis. Cartilage 2017;8(4):374–83.

18. Ng A, Bernhard A, Bernhard K. Advances in ankle cartilage repair. Clin Podiatr Med Surg 2017;34(4):471–87.

19. Shieh AK, Singh SG, Nathe C, et al. Effects of micronized cartilage matrix on cartilage repair in osteochondral lesions of the talus. Cartilage 2020;11(3): 316–22.

20. Allahabadi S, Johnson B, Whitney M, et al. Short-term outcomes following dehydrated micronized allogenic cartilage versus isolated microfracture for treatment of medial talar osteochondral lesions. Foot Ankle Surg 2022;28(5):642–9.

21. Riff AJ, Davey A, Cole BJ. Emerging technologies in cartilage restoration. In: Yanke A, Cole B, editors. Joint preservation of the knee. Cham: Springer; 2019. https://doi.org/10.1007/978-3-030-01491-9_18.

22. Beth ZC, Sachs B, Kruse D, et al. Arthroscopic implantation of a cartilage matrix for an osteochondral defect of the talus: a case report. J Foot Ankle Surg 2019; 58(5):1014–8.

23. Yontar NS, Aslan L, Öğüt T. Functional outcomes of autologous matrix-related chondrogenesis to treat large osteochondral lesions of the talus. Foot Ankle Int 2022;43(6):783–9.

24. Fortier LA, Barker JU, Strauss EJ, et al. The role of growth factors in cartilage repair. Clin Orthop Relat Res 2011;469(10):2706–15.

25. Chahla J, Cinque ME, Shon JM, et al. Bone marrow aspirate concentrate for the treatment of osteochondral lesions of the talus: a systematic review of outcomes. J Exp Orthop 2016;3(1):33 [Erratum in: J Exp Orthop. 2016 Dec;3(1):38. PMID: 27813021; PMCID: PMC5095091].

26. Fortier LA, Nixon AJ, Williams J, et al. Isolation and chondrocytic differentiation of equine bone marrow-derived mesenchymal stem cells. Am J Vet Res 1998;59(9): 1182–7.

27. Drakos MC, Hansen OB, Eble SK, et al. Augmenting osteochondral autograft transplantation and bone marrow aspirate concentrate with particulate cartilage extracellular matrix is associated with improved outcomes. Foot Ankle Int 2022; 43(9):1131–42.

28. Vannini F, Filardo G, Altamura SA, et al. Bone marrow aspirate concentrate and scaffold for osteochondral lesions of the talus in ankle osteoarthritis: satisfactory clinical outcome at 10 years. Knee Surg Sports Traumatol Arthrosc 2021;29(8): 2504–10.

29. Grigolo B, Lisignoli G, Piacentini A, et al. Evidence for redifferentiation of human chondrocytes grown on a hyaluronan-based biomaterial (HYAff 11): molecular, immunohistochemical and ultrastructural analysis. Biomaterials 2002;23(4): 1187–95.

30. Sadlik B, Gobbi A, Puszkarz M, et al. Biologic inlay osteochondral reconstruction: arthroscopic one-step osteochondral lesion repair in the knee using morselized bone grafting and hyaluronic acid-based scaffold embedded with bone marrow aspirate concentrate. Arthrosc Tech 2017;6(2):e383-9.
31. Gobbi A, Whyte GP. One-Stage cartilage repair using a hyaluronic acid-based scaffold with activated bone marrow-derived mesenchymal stem cells compared with microfracture: five-year follow-up. Am J Sports Med 2016;44(11):2846-54.

Arthroscopic Lateral Stabilization

Joseph Wolf, DPM, AACFAS[a], James Cottom, DPM[b], Jonathon Srour, DPM, AACFAS[c], Laurence Rubin, DPM[d],*

KEYWORDS

- Sprain • Reconstruction • Arthroscopy • Ankle joint • Subtalar joint
- Anterior talofibular ligament • Calcaneal fibular ligament • Stabilization

KEY POINTS

- Arthroscopic modified Brostrom repair has shown equivalent passive range of motion and biomechanical outcomes to open repair through a smaller incision.
- The arthroscopic approach allows for other procedures including repair of osteochondral lesions (OCL) through the same incisions.
- There are less reported complications with the arthroscopic approach versus open.

INTRODUCTION

The ankle is one of the most common traumatized bodily areas in sports representing up to 30% of all injuries.[1–4] Of the reported injuries, up to 77%[5] involve the lateral ankle and 73% involve tearing or rupture of the anterior talofibular ligament (ATFL).[6] Following the initial sprain 70% of individuals report at least one recurrent ankle sprain[4] with up to 40% developing chronic lateral ankle instability.[7]

Initial treatment is based on severity and often involves a combination of offloading, anti-inflammatories, ice, and progressive mobilization and physical therapy. It has been reported that 80% to 85% of acute ankle sprains respond well to functional rehabilitation programs with the remainder suffering recurrent instability.[8] For those who fail conservative management ankle instability is surgically treated. The goal of surgery is to: decrease pain, restore stability to the ankle, restore proprioception, allow for return to activity, and prevent accelerated arthritis.

Since Brostrom[9] first described an anatomic lateral ankle ligament repair in 1966 there have been many modifications to the original procedure. Most notably was the

[a] Florida Orthopedic Foot and Ankle Center, 4913 Harroun Road, Suite 1, Sylvania, OH 43560, USA; [b] Florida Orthopedic Foot and Ankle Center Fellowship, 5741 Bee Ridge Road, Suite 490, Sarasota, Fl 34233, USA; [c] Virginia Fellowship in Reconstruction, Revision, and Limb Preservation Surgery of the Foot and Ankle, 905 South Willow Avenue, Cookeville, TN 38501, USA; [d] Virginia Fellowship in Reconstruction, Revision, and Limb Preservation Surgery of the Foot and Ankle, 7016 Lee Park Road, Suite 105, Mechanicsville, VA 23111, USA
* Corresponding author.
E-mail address: lgrubin1413@gmail.com

Clin Podiatr Med Surg 40 (2023) 495–507
https://doi.org/10.1016/j.cpm.2023.03.002
0891-8422/23/© 2023 Elsevier Inc. All rights reserved.

Gould modification adding the inferior extensor retinaculum in 1980.[10] Today the same tissue is used with the added strength of different types and combinations of anchors. In 2011 Acevedo and Mangone[11] described an all inside arthroscopic approach to lateral ankle stabilization. The arthroscopic approach allowed for complete visualization of the ankle joint itself, and allowed for repair with minimal soft tissue dissection. Odak and coworkers[12] in 2015 found with chronic lateral instability 63% of patients had synovitis, 17% had osteochondral lesions, and 12% suffered from ankle impingement, which is not routinely visualized through the open approach. Although the arthroscopic Brostrom procedure has undergone multiple modifications, in this article we present the author's preferred approach. Early studies showed a positive diagnostic and therapeutic benefit to the patient for arthroscopy directly before the open incision required for the ankle stabilization procedures. Thus, arthroscopy is currently advocated as an adjunct procedure before an open or mini-open stabilization procedure. One should note that this evolution of open procedure, to arthroscopy plus an open procedure is similar to the history of stabilization procedures in the knee and shoulder before completely arthroscopic procedures becoming the standard of care for those joints.

PREOPERATIVE WORK-UP

As with any surgical procedure, the correct diagnosis is vital to a successful arthroscopic stabilization. Instability can create secondary pathology in the joint. When performing a preoperative evaluation for instability it is important to identify which structures are involved. The surgeon needs to determine if this is a single or double ligament injury, what joints are involved (ankle and/or subtalar joints), and any secondary pathology.

Anterior drawer and talar tilt determine which ligaments are affected. The palpatory examination determines if the pathology is in the ankle joint or both the ankle and subtalar joints. Selective blocks of the joints is used to help isolate which joints are involved. The authors of the arthroscopic double ligament stabilization consider doing a single joint (ankle) arthroscopic ligament stabilization when only the ATFL and only the ankle joint are involved on examination.

Through comparative palpation, neighboring anatomic structures are effectively ruled out as contributory to the patient's pain. These include the peroneal tendons, deltoid ligament, calcaneal-cuboid joint, and talonavicular joint.

Advanced imaging is recommended in the case of recurrent and chronic lateral ankle instability. In addition to the ability to assess the lateral ankle ligaments themselves, MRI can provide further insight on the tibiofibular/syndesmotic ligaments and the talus itself for osteochondral lesions, which may also be addressed at the time of surgery.

ARTHROSCOPIC MODIFIED BROSTROM PROCEDURE FOR LATERAL ANKLE INSTABILITY
Surgical Technique

This procedure is performed using the standard ankle arthroscopic anterior approach. Initially the medial and lateral malleoli, peroneal and tibialis anterior tendons, and intermediate dorsal cutaneous nerve (IDCN) are mapped out followed by establishing the medial and lateral portals. Four points are then marked equidistant from one another in an arc between the IDCN and the peroneal tendons 1.5 to 2 cm distal to the tip of the fibula (**Fig. 1**). Once the portals are established the ankle joint is then debrided in its entirety. Following debridement, the talar dome and the tibial plafond are visually inspected. The anterior face of the lateral malleoli is then debrided using a shaver

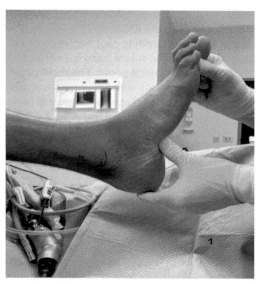

Fig. 1. Four points are marked equidistant from one another in an arc between the IDCN and the peroneal tendons 1.5 to 2 cm distal to the tip of the fibula.

initially followed by an ablator to allow complete visualization. It is necessary to adequately expose the malleolus to allow for direct bony visualization and anchor placement. A drill guide is placed through the anterolateral portal with the trocar in place and used to visualize the medial, lateral, and distal borders of the fibula. The guide is then positioned 1 cm proximal to the distal fibular tip and centered on the malleolus. The fibula is drilled, and a double loaded 3.0-mm anchor is inserted (**Fig. 2**). The two suture arms from the anchor are then passed through the anterolateral portal. To capture the ATFL and inferior extensor retinaculum we prefer the "outside-in"

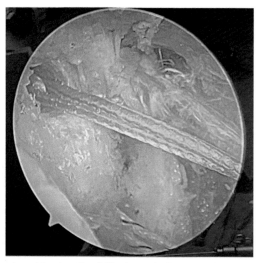

Fig. 2. First anchor placed in the distal fibula with the second anchor at the level of the ankle joint.

technique wherein a microsuture lasso is percutaneously inserted into each of the four previously marked points between the IDCN and the peroneal tendons (**Fig. 3**). The lasso must be passed at adequate depth to capture the inferior extensor retinaculum, ATFL, and the ankle joint capsule. The suture lasso is inserted in the most posterior of the four points (point 1) exiting the lateral portal. The most proximal suture is looped through the lasso and passed exiting the skin. This process is repeated for the second suture (point 2). A second anchor is then placed at the level of the talar dome in the central face of the fibula. The second anchor's suture arms are then routed in the same manner as the first anchor with the most proximal suture arm exiting point 4 (see **Fig. 3**). A small incision is then made between sutures 2 and 3 bluntly dissecting down to the inferior extensor retinaculum (IER). A bluntly hooked probe is inserted subcutaneously and superficial to the IER and is used to pull each of the sutures into the accessory incision while maintaining anchor integrity (**Fig. 4**). The noninvasive ankle distracter is released, the ankle is held in maximum dorsiflexion and eversion, and the sutures are hand tied again maintaining anchor integrity (**Fig. 5**). An accessory incision is then made lateral to the distal fibula in the midline of the fibula 3 cm proximal to the fibular tip. A suture lasso is then passed subperiosteally exiting at the connecting incision between the suture points (**Fig. 6**). The tails of the tied suture are then grasped and passed back to the fibula. The lateral face of the fibula is drilled, and the suture tails are passed through a 2.9-mm anchor (**Fig. 7**). With the ankle maintained in further dorsiflexion and eversion the suture anchor is then inserted. The remainder of the suture are then cut. Anterior drawer and inversion stress examinations are completed to confirm adequate stabilization. The incisions are then closed in standard fashion. The patient is then placed in a tall leg controlled ankle motion boot and instructed to remain nonweightbearing for 24 hours after which they are permitted assisted weightbearing as tolerated with crutches. At 2 weeks the sutures are removed with therapy started at Week 3. At Week 4 the patient is transitioned out of the boot and into an ankle brace while the remainder of therapy is completed. Patients remain in the brace for day-to-day activity for 3 months, after which they use the brace for rigorous activity only. Patients are typically without the brace full time by 6 months postoperatively.

Procedure Pearls

Although the procedure itself is straightforward the author has a few technique tips to ensure smooth execution. The importance of a thorough debridement cannot be

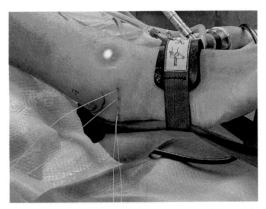

Fig. 3. Suture from the most distal anchor exiting spots 1 and 2 and the most proximal anchor suture exiting spots 3 and 4.

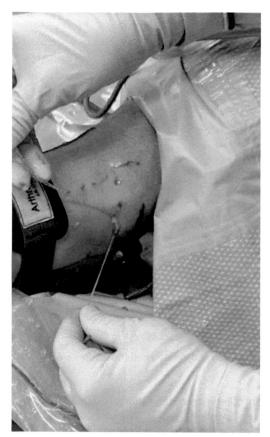

Fig. 4. An incision is made between sutures 2 and 3 with all four sutures being gathered in the middle.

stressed enough, and the entire anterior face of the lateral malleolus must be visualized to ensure the anchors capture the fibula and do not exit the lateral cortex. Once the anchors are inserted (while visualizing the anchor with the scope) pull on one of the suture arms to differentiate between proximal and distal suture arms. It is also beneficial to use different pattern sutures to maintain anchor integrity (ie, tiger stripe and solid color suture). When tying the suture, with the foot maintained in slight dorsiflexion and eversion the suture arms need only be tied with moderated tension and one should avoid pistoning the individual suture arms because this creates a sawing motion and can cut the soft tissue and cause loss of correction. When passing the suture ensure there is adequate slack for the suture to reach its destination. The accessory incision can also be modified to allow for peroneal tendon inspection and repair if need be, without a separate incision.

Biomechanical Data

The lateral ankle complex consists of the ATFL, calcaneofibular ligament, and posterior talofibular ligament. The ATFL is the weakest and most often torn ligament with an ultimate load to failure of 138 to 160 N.[13] Drakos and coworkers[14] in 2014 performed a biomechanical comparison of open versus arthroscopic lateral ankle reconstruction

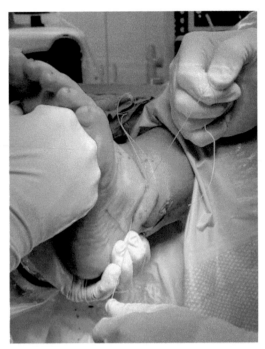

Fig. 5. The foot is dorsiflexed and everted and the sutures are hand tied maintaining anchor integrity.

finding no significant difference in translation of the talus in all planes between the two techniques. Lee and coworkers[15] in 2016 also performed biomechanical testing of open versus arthroscopic modified Brostrom using a single anchor, whereas Drakos used a two-anchor construct. Lee's study similarly found no significance between the two in torque to failure, degrees to failure, and stiffness.[15] Cottom and coworkers[16] in 2016 compared three different arthroscopic techniques finding a three-anchor construct as the most stable with a maximum load of 246.82 ± 82.37, as was presented in this article.

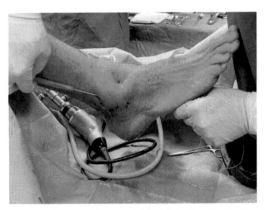

Fig. 6. After the suture is tied a suture passer is passed subperiosteally drawing all four sutures to the distal fibula.

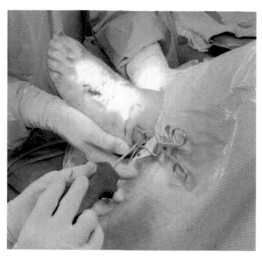

Fig. 7. The sutures are then anchored into the fibula.

Outcomes Data

Cottom and colleagues[17] reported on 45 patients with an average follow-up of 14 months following arthroscopic Brostrom repair with the additional anchor as described previously. At 1 year the average American Orthopedic Foot and Ankle Society (AOFAS) scores improved from 48.7 preoperatively to 95.4 postoperatively. Visual analog scores also decreased from 8 preoperatively to 0.9 postoperatively. Yeo and colleagues[18] reported on 28 patients using two knotless anchors in the fibula and found improvement in the AOFAS score to 89 and decrease in the VAS score to 2. **Table 1** provides a summary of recent publications. When compared with open repair, the arthroscopic Brostrom outperformed open repair in postoperative AOFAS scores, VAS scores, and time to weightbearing with comparable operative time.[19] Complication rates have also been lower in the arthroscopic groups with rates of 6.5% compared with 11.1% in open group.[17]

Summary

Arthroscopic modified Brostrom procedure creates a strong repair with minimal soft tissue dissection. Although there is a learning curve with this procedure, it is a reliable, minimally invasive approach to lateral ankle stabilization. In addition to smaller incisions, this approach allows for ankle joint debridement and inspection of the articular surfaces without requiring an open arthrotomy. Treatment of osteochondral lesions can also be performed concomitantly again without further dissection. This technique is a minimally invasive approach to lateral ankle stabilization with no statistically significant biomechanical differences, lower complication rates, and faster return to activity. The arthroscopic modified Brostrom is becoming the gold standard for primary repair of lateral ankle instability.

ARTHROSCOPIC DOUBLE LIGAMENT STABILIZATION
Positioning

The arthroscopic double ligament stabilization procedure is performed with the patient supine on table. An ipsilateral hip bump is used for internal rotation. An additional bump underneath the ipsilateral foot/leg may sometimes be required for optimum

Table 1
Summary of literature on functional outcomes following arthroscopic Brostrum repair

Author, Year	Level of Evidence	No. of Ankles	No. of Anchors	Follow-up	Preoperative AOFAS	Postoperative AOFAS	Satisfaction Rate (%)
Corte-Real & Moreira,[20] 2009	IV, retrospective case series	28	2	27.5 mo (6–48 mo)	—	85.3 (65–100)	NA
Cottom & Rigby,[21] 2013	IV, case series	40	2	12.13 mo (6–21 mo)	41.2	95.4 (84–100)	NA
Kim et al,[22] 2011	IV, retrospective case series	28	2	15.9 mo (13–25 mo)	60.78	92.48	—
Labib & Slone,[23] 2015	IV, retrospective case series	14	2	3 mo (6–54 wk)	NA	92.8 (80–100)	86
Li et al,[24] 2017	III, retrospective cohort	23	1 or 2	39.7 mo	69.3	93.3	—
Nery et al,[25] 2011	IV, retrospective case series	38	2	9.8 y (5–14 y)	NA	90 (44–100)	94.7
Nery et al,[26] 2018	II, prospective cohort	26	1	27 mo (21–36 mo)	58	90	NA
Song et al,[27] 2017	III, retrospective cohort	16	1	16.3 mo	59.3	93	—
Vega et al,[28] 2013	IV, retrospective case series	16	1	22.3 mo (12–35 mo)	67	97 (95–100)	NA
Yeo et al,[28] 2016	I, randomized control trial	25	1	NA	67.5	90.3	—
Cottom et al,[17] 2016	III, retrospective cohort	45	3	14 mo[12–17,19,20]	48.7	95.4 (90–100)	—

Abbreviations: NA, not applicable or not mentioned.

access to the subtalar joint portals. A thigh tourniquet is applied but rarely inflated. An ankle distractor is never used unless a concomitant procedure involving a repair of an osteochondral lesion is necessary. The portals of the ankle and the subtalar joints are marked before insufflation to avoid losing the bony landmarks. Approximately 10 mL of 0.5% Marcaine with epinephrine is injected into each joint taking care to withdraw slowly to provide hemostatic effect to the portals themselves.

Surgical Technique

Standard portals of the ankle and the subtalar joints are established. A 4.0-mm, 70° scope is traditionally used but smaller diameter and 30° arthroscopes can also be used. A combination of a sucker shaver and thermal ablation is used to remove synovitis, scar tissue, and impingement lesions. The cartilage is inspected for any defects or lesions. A thorough debridement of the medial aspect of the joint provides a clear medial viewing portal. The lateral aspect of the ankle and the lateral gutter are debrided while preserving the ATFL (**Fig. 8**). The lateral aspect of the fibula is prepared for the Brostrom by debriding the cortex with an arthroscopic burr.

The distal fibula is drilled and tapped (**Figs. 9–12**) and a 4.5-mm anchor is inserted with a 1.6-mm suture tape and a 2.0 suture attached to it. The lateral talus is then drilled and tapped for a 3.5 knotless anchor, with attention given to aiming away from the subtalar joint. The arthroscopic instrumentation is removed from the ankle and the subtalar joint is entered with the standard lateral portal used as a viewing portal and the anterolateral portal used as the working portal.

The subtalar joint is debrided and the lateral wall of the calcaneus is drilled and tapped for a 3.5-mm knotless anchor (**Fig. 10A**). An arthroscopic suture grasper is placed from the subtalar joint into the ankle. One of the two arms of the suture tape from the 4.5 anchor in the fibula is grasped and brought into the subtalar joint (**Fig. 11**). Once the arm of the suture tape is in the subtalar joint, it is inserted into the calcaneus with a 3.5 knotless anchor, while holding the subtalar joint in eversion (**Fig. 10B**).

The arthroscopic instrumentation is removed from the subtalar joint and the ankle joint is reentered with the anteromedial portal once again the viewing portal and the anterolateral portal the working portal. The remaining arm of the suture tape is placed into the talus with a 3.5 knotless anchor while the ankle is held in 90° and eversion (**Fig. 12**). A single ligament stabilization of the ATFL is performed by eliminating the subtalar portion of the procedure and placing both arms of the suture tape from the fibula into the talus.

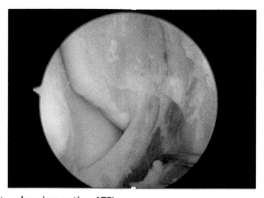

Fig. 8. Lateral gutter showing native ATFL.

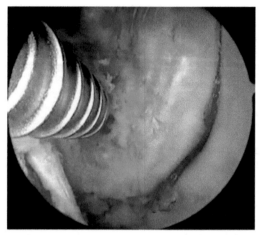

Fig. 9. Drilling for 4.5-mm fibular anchor.

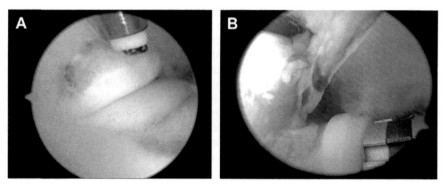

Fig. 10. Arthroscopic debridement of the subtalar joint. (*A*) arthroscopic debridement of the subtalar joint; (*B*) insertion of a 3.5mm knotless anchor into the calcaneus through the subtalar joint portals.

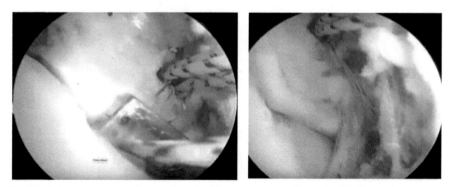

Fig. 11. Suture grasper with one strand of the suture tape from the fibular anchor.

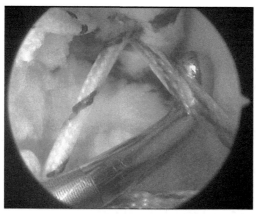

Fig. 12. Reconstructed double ligament (*blue tape*) with Brostrum (*black/white suture*).

The Brostrom is performed by using a suture passer to grab the lateral capsule from the inside of the ankle joint. A Tennessee slider knot secures the capsule down to the distal fibula that had previously been prepared with the arthroscopic burr. This creates an arthroscopic Brostrom and helps restore proprioception to the joint. The portals are closed in standard fashion and a well-padded posterior splint is applied.

Postoperative Care

The patient is kept in a posterior splint for 3 weeks at which point they are advanced to weightbearing as tolerated in a CAM boot for an additional 2 weeks. At 6 weeks postoperatively, they are advanced to weightbearing as tolerated in normal shoe wear.

SUMMARY

Arthroscopic double ligament stabilization procedure creates a robust reconstruction of the anterior talofibular and calcaneal fibular ligaments with minimal soft tissue dissection. Although this is a technically challenging procedure, it minimizes scar tissue and trauma to the soft tissues. Much like the evolution of shoulder and knee arthroscopic procedures, this procedure is now truly arthroscopic without the need for ancillary portals or additional incisions. Treatment of osteochondral lesions can also be performed concomitantly again without further dissection. The arthroscopic double ligament stabilization may be the future of ankle and hindfoot stabilization procedures.

DISCLOSURES

J. Srour has nothing to disclose. L. Rubin is a consultant for Parcus and Vilex. J. Wolf has nothing to disclose. J. Cottom is a consultant for Arthrex, Naples, FL.

REFERENCES

1. Holmer P, Sondergaard L, Konradsen L, et al. Epidemiology of sprains in the lateral ankle and foot. Foot Ankle Int 1994;15(2):72–4.
2. Garrick JG, Requa RK. The epidemiology of foot and ankle injuries in sports. Clin Sports Med 1988;7(1):29–36.
3. MacAuley D. Ankle injuries: same joint, different sports. Med Sci Sports Exerc 1999;31(7 Suppl):S409–11.

4. Yeung MS, Chan KM, So CH, et al. An epidemiological survey on ankle sprain. Br J Sports Med 1994;28(2):112–6.
5. Fong DT, Hong Y, Chan LK, et al. A systematic review on ankle injury and ankle sprain in sports. Sports Med 2007;37(1):73–94. https://doi.org/10.2165/00007256-200737010-00006.
6. Gerber JP, Williams GN, Scoville CR, et al. Persistent disability associated with ankle sprains: a prospective examination of an athletic population. Foot Ankle Int 1998;19(10):653–60.
7. Woods C, Hawkins R, Hulse M, et al. The Football Association Medical Research Programme: an audit of injuries in professional football. An analysis of ankle sprains. Br J Sports Med 2003;37(3):233–8.
8. Baumhauer JF, O'Brien T. Surgical considerations in the treatment of ankle instability. J Athl Train 2002;37(4):458–62.
9. Broström L. Sprained ankles. VI. Surgical treatment of "chronic" ligament ruptures. Acta Chir Scand 1966;132(5):551–65.
10. Gould N, Seligson D, Gassman J. Early and late repair of lateral ligament of the ankle. Foot Ankle 1980;1(2):84–9.
11. Acevedo J, Mangone P. Arthroscopic lateral ankle ligament reconstruction. Tech Foot Ankle Surg 2011;10:111–6.
12. Odak S, Ahluwalia R, Shivarathre DG, et al. Arthroscopic evaluation of impingement and osteochondral lesions in chronic lateral ankle instability. Foot Ankle Int 2015;36(9):1045–9.
13. Viens NA, Wijdicks CA, Campbell KJ, et al. Anterior talofibular ligament ruptures, part 1: biomechanical comparison of augmented Broström repair techniques with the intact anterior talofibular ligament. Am J Sports Med 2014;42(2):405–11.
14. Drakos MC, Behrens SB, Paller D, et al. Biomechanical comparison of an open vs arthroscopic approach for lateral ankle instability. Foot Ankle Int 2014;35(8):809–15.
15. Lee KT, Kim ES, Kim YH, et al. All-inside arthroscopic modified Broström operation for chronic ankle instability: a biomechanical study. Knee Surg Sports Traumatol Arthrosc 2016;24(4):1096–100.
16. Cottom JM, Baker JS, Richardson PE, et al. A biomechanical comparison of 3 different arthroscopic lateral ankle stabilization techniques in 36 cadaveric ankles. J Foot Ankle Surg 2016;55(6):1229–33.
17. Cottom JM, Baker JS, Richardson PE. The "all-inside" arthroscopic Broström procedure with additional suture anchor augmentation: a prospective study of 45 consecutive patients. J Foot Ankle Surg 2016;55(6):1223–8.
18. Yeo ED, Lee KT, Sung IH, et al. Comparison of all-inside arthroscopic and open techniques for the modified Broström procedure for ankle instability. Foot Ankle Int 2016;37(10):1037–45.
19. Zhou YF, Zhang ZZ, Zhang HZ, et al. All-inside arthroscopic modified Broström technique to repair anterior talofibular ligament provides a similar outcome compared with open Broström-Gould procedure. Arthroscopy 2021;37(1):268–79.
20. Corte-Real NM, Moreira RM. Arthroscopic repair of chronic lateral ankle instability. Foot Ankle Int 2009;30(3):213–7.
21. Cottom JM, Rigby RB. The "all inside" arthroscopic Broström procedure: a prospective study of 40 consecutive patients. J Foot Ankle Surg 2013;52(5):568–74.
22. Kim ES, Lee KT, Park JS, et al. Arthroscopic anterior talofibular ligament repair for chronic ankle instability with a suture anchor technique. Orthopedics 2011;34(4). https://doi.org/10.3928/01477447-20110228-03.

23. Labib SA, Slone HS. Ankle arthroscopy for lateral ankle instability. Tech Foot Ankle Surg 2015;14(1):25–7.

24. Li H, Hua Y, Li H, et al. Activity level and function 2 years after anterior talofibular ligament repair: a comparison between arthroscopic repair and open repair procedures. Am J Sports Med 2017;45(9):2044–51.

25. Nery C, Raduan F, Del Buono A, et al. Arthroscopic-assisted Broström-Gould for chronic ankle instability: a long-term follow-up. Am J Sports Med 2011;39(11): 2381–8.

26. Nery C, Fonseca L, Raduan F, et al, ESSKA AFAS Ankle Instability Group. Prospective study of the " inside-out" arthroscopic ankle ligament technique: preliminary result. Foot Ankle Surg 2018;24(4):320–5.

27. Song B, Li C, Chen N, et al. All-arthroscopic anatomical reconstruction of anterior talofibular ligament using semitendinosus autografts. Int Orthop 2017;41(5): 975–82.

28. Vega J, Golanó P, Pellegrino A, et al. All-inside arthroscopic lateral collateral ligament repair for ankle instability with a knotless suture anchor technique. Foot Ankle Int 2013;34(12):1701–9.

The Role of Arthroscopy After Total Ankle Replacement

Lawrence DiDomenico, DPM[a,b,]*, John A. Martucci, DPM[a],
Samantha A. Miner, DPM[c]

KEYWORDS

- Total ankle arthroplasty • TAR • Arthroscopy • Impingement • Gutter pain

KEY POINTS

- Arthroscopy is a valuable tool for assessment and treatment of pain owing to impingement after total ankle arthroplasty.
- If no other procedures are indicated, then arthroscopy can be a successful treatment to get patients back to painless activity quickly.
- An open arthrotomy is advised for the inexperienced arthroscopist, as damage to the prosthesis components could be detrimental.

INTRODUCTION

Alongside advances and trends in foot and ankle surgery, arthroscopy provides a minimally invasive option for exploring and addressing pain after total ankle replacement (TAR). As literature purports, TAR is not without its complications. Procedure execution and outcomes can be variable, from wound-healing issues and infection, to aseptic loosening and implant failure.[1] Furthermore, reoperation rates after TAR are higher than its primary alternative, ankle arthrodesis.[2] However, as implant design and surgeon experience improve, so too does implant survivorship.[3,4] The total ankle surgeon must understand the variety of complications that may arise and how best to manage them to preserve implant longevity.

It is not uncommon for patients to develop pain months or even years after TAR. A systematic review by Gougoulias and colleagues[5] in 2010 found a rate of 27% to 60% of residual pain after TAR at greater than 2 years follow-up among a variety of implants. One common cause of residual pain after TAR is impingement. The incidence

[a] Reconstructive Rearfoot and Ankle Fellowship, NOMS Ankle and Foot Care Center, 8175 Market Street, Youngstown, OH 44512, USA; [b] East Liverpool City Hospital Residency Program, East Liverpool, OH, USA; [c] Reconstructive Foot and Ankle Fellowship, Coordinated Health/ Lehigh Valley Health Network, 2774 Schoenersville Road, Bethlehem, PA 18017, USA
* Corresponding author. 8175 Market Street, Youngstown, OH 44512.
E-mail address: LD5353@aol.com

Clin Podiatr Med Surg 40 (2023) 509–518
https://doi.org/10.1016/j.cpm.2023.03.003   podiatric.theclinics.com
0891-8422/23/© 2023 Elsevier Inc. All rights reserved.

of pain owing to impingement has been reported to be as high as 45%.[6] This condition can be either soft tissue or osseous in nature. It results in a chronic inflammatory reaction within the joint leading to pain as well as reduced motion or abnormal function.[7]

The most common location for impingement after TAR is the anteromedial ankle. Factors that can lead to impingement include improper implant position or size, component loosening, type of prosthesis, residual varus/valgus deformity, insufficient gutter debridement, and soft tissue imbalance. [6,8] There is also a small subset of patients that may present without any clear underlying cause for impingement.[9,10] In these cases, it is typically a diagnosis of exclusion.

Traditionally, impingement in patients with TAR has been treated through an open arthrotomy. However, more recently, arthroscopic debridement has been proposed as an alternative to the open procedure. The benefits of arthroscopy include its minimally invasive approach, faster recovery and return to function, and decreased risk of wound dehiscence, scar tissue formation, and periprosthetic joint infection. If a patient's symptoms can be attributed to bony or soft tissue impingement alone, arthroscopy can serve as a valuable diagnostic and treatment tool. However, if one of the aforementioned factors is contributing to impingement, then additional procedures may be required, and arthroscopy may be used adjunctively. This article serves as an introduction to the utilization of arthroscopy after TAR.

INDICATIONS FOR ARTHROSCOPY AFTER A TOTAL ANKLE REPLACEMENT

Proper evaluation of the cause of residual pain after TAR, and whether arthroscopy is indicated, is heavily reliant on history and physical examination. Index of suspicion for impingement should be raised in a patient with uncomplicated TAR that presents with persistent postoperative pain—particularly on exertion, edema localized to the ankle, and ankle gutter tenderness. In the case of soft tissue impingement, radiographs will be otherwise normal. Osseous impingement from heterotopic bone is often more straightforward to identify, because this can often be visualized on radiographs or computed tomography (CT). The most common osseous impingement occurs between the prosthesis and the malleoli. Conservative measures, including physical therapy, injections, and foot orthoses, should be attempted before any surgical intervention.[11,12]

For uncomplicated TARs that do not require concomitant procedures, arthroscopic debridement can be considered if conservative measures fail. Patients should be educated preoperatively on the need to possibly convert to open arthrotomy as well as the possibility of additional revision procedures in the future. Common indications for arthroscopic debridement after TAR are a minimum of 90 days after implantation, isolated pain to the medial and/or lateral ankle gutters, heterotopic bone present on radiographs, or pain with exertion without any other evident cause on radiographs. Contraindications include prosthesis loosening or periprosthetic joint infection, as these issues require alternative approaches and would be inadequately addressed with arthroscopy. A summary of the indications and contraindications for arthroscopic debridement after TAR is represented in **Table 1**. [8,9,13,14]

Other contraindications to arthroscopy include the presence of significant heterotopic bone or the need for polyethylene exchange owing to accelerated wear. In these types of situations, an open arthrotomy is advised.[15]

Additional considerations before arthroscopic intervention include the possible need for concomitant procedures to address the factors predisposing the patient to impingement. For instance, if the patient has an undercorrected varus deformity resulting in medial ankle impingement, a lateralizing calcaneal osteotomy may be

Table 1 Indication and contraindications for arthroscopy after total ankle replacement	
Indications	**Contraindications**
>90 d after TAR implantation	Periprosthetic joint infection
Focal tenderness to medial and/or lateral gutters	Prosthesis loosening or subsidence requiring revision
Heterotopic bone formation at the prosthesis-malleolar interface on radiographs or CT	Need for concomitant open procedures (eg, polyethylene exchange)
OR pain with exertion *without* any other evident cause on radiographs	Severe heterotopic bone formation

necessary in addition to arthroscopic debridement. This serves to decompress the medial gutter and restore biomechanical balance. Although discussion of these concomitant procedures is beyond the scope of this article, the surgeon must be aware of all possible causes for pain after TAR.[8,11]

SURGICAL APPROACHES FOR ARTHROSCOPY AFTER TOTAL ANKLE REPLACEMENT
Anterior Approach

For access to the medial and lateral gutters, an anterior approach is advised using the standard anteromedial and anterolateral portals for arthroscopy of the ankle. The anteromedial portal is placed medial to the tibialis anterior tendon at the anterior ankle joint line. The anterolateral portal is placed just lateral to the peroneus tertius tendon (or extensor digitorum longus tendon if peroneus tertius is absent) at the anterior ankle joint line.

Controversy exists regarding the use of ankle distraction. Distraction may improve both visualization and ease of procedure, although this is largely up to the surgeon's preference. The type of arthroscope to use for this procedure also varies based on surgeon preference. A 2.7- or 4.0-mm arthroscope with a 30° camera is typically used for standard ankle arthroscopy. However, a 70° angled camera can provide a larger field of view and enables the arthroscopist to peek around corners. This allows greater visual access to the deeper aspects of the medial and lateral gutters. It is the authors' preference to use a 4.0-mm 30° arthroscope without distraction. The authors believe this provides the appropriate amount of visualization to allow for adequate debridement of the ankle gutters.

The presence of dense, fibrotic scar tissue within the soft tissues of the anterior ankle can make the arthroscopic portals more difficult to establish. As a result, placing the ankle in full dorsiflexion is recommended during initial penetration of the capsule in order to protect the prosthesis, particularly the talar component, from damage. Once the camera is inserted, it should be noted that the metallic components are highly reflective. This results in a mirror image effect that can be disorienting. Orientation can be achieved by touching the shaver to the scope and repeating this with the remaining structures within the joint. A 3.5-mm shaver is typically used initially for debridement. It is advised to keep the blunt or hooded end of the shaver in contact with the prosthesis in order to prevent scratching of the components. A burr, small curette, or bipolar radiofrequency ablator may also be used for removal of fibrotic soft tissue and heterotopic bone. [8,11]

In a retrospective review by Kim and colleagues,[9] residual pain after TAR was most commonly present in the medial gutter. For debridement of the medial gutter, one should place the arthroscope in the anterolateral portal, with the working instrument in the medial portal. The shaver, or other debridement tool, should be oriented as close to parallel to the medial gutter as possible. Adequate decompression of the gutter is achieved when the posterior tibial tendon can be visualized. Debridement should be performed carefully, because aggressive and over-debridement can result in fracture of the medial malleolus.[13,14,16,17]

Debridement of the lateral gutter is similar to that of the medial gutter. The arthroscope is placed within the anteromedial portal, while the shaver or other instrument is placed within the anterolateral portal. While working in the lateral gutter, the arthroscopist must remain close to talus to prevent overresection of fibula. A sufficient amount of debridement has been performed when the peroneal tendons are able to be visualized. [13–15]

Fluoroscopy is often recommended once debridement has concluded in order to verify that no further bony impingement remains. Aside from weight-bearing radiographs preoperatively, placing a patient through range of motion while under anesthesia also allows the surgeon to recognize potential areas of impingement.[14]

Posterior approach

The incidence of heterotopic ossification after TAR is more than 70% and most commonly affects the posterior aspect of the ankle joint.[18,19] However, bony overgrowth in the posterior ankle is often asymptomatic in patients with TAR, even when radiographic evidence is present. Arthroscopic intervention should only be undertaken in symptomatic patients. Furthermore, if a patient presents with large amounts of posterior heterotopic bone, an open arthrotomy should also be considered.

Distraction for a posterior approach is often difficult and is not routinely used. When performing a posterior debridement in combination with an anterior approach, an anterior posteromedial (just anterior to the posterior tibial tendon) and posterolateral (just posterior to the peroneal tendons) portal can be used. This would be an ideal approach for cases of posterior soft tissue impingement.

However, in cases of heterotopic ossification within the posterior aspect of the joint, a prone position is preferred. The posterolateral portal is made at the level of the distal tip of the fibula and just lateral to the Achilles tendon. The posteromedial portal is made at the same level just medial to the Achilles tendon. Fluoroscopy may be useful to identify the joint line, because this can often be obscured by heterotopic bone posteriorly. Care should be taken to avoid damaging the flexor hallucis longus tendon, as well as the neurovascular structures medially with this approach. Bone debridement can be performed with an arthroscopic rongeur or punch, such as the Ferris-Smith Kerrison rongeur. A small burr or curette can also be used in these cases.[7,8]

A CASE STUDY

This patient presented with a painful right ankle. He has had no significant past medical history. He was involved in an automobile accident approximately 15 years before presenting to the authors' clinic and sustained severe ankle injury to his right ankle. He developed debilitating posttraumatic osteoarthritis and subsequently underwent a lateral approach ankle fusion with an outside provider (**Figs. 1A–C and 2**). Unfortunately, the attempted ankle fusion went on to a painful nonunion of the tibial talar joint. He was experiencing constant aches and intermittent shooting pains with ambulation and was seeking reevaluation by a different foot and ankle surgeon. Given the failed attempted arthrodesis, a TAR was suggested. He underwent a surgical procedure consisting of removal of existing hardware, a lateral approach TAR. Months following implantation, he experienced a syndesmosis nonunion and pain in the lateral gutter and persistent discomfort with ambulation (**Fig. 3A**).

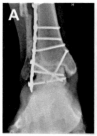
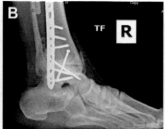
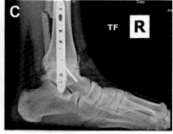

Fig. 1. (*A–C*) Pre-Operative anteroposterior (AP), medial oblique, and lateral preoperative radiographs demonstrating broken hardware (*A*) and a nonunion of the fibula (*B*) and the tibial talar joint (*C*).

A revision surgery consisted of a repair of the syndesmosis nonunion and an ankle joint arthroscopy to explore and debride tissue along the medial and lateral gutters (**Figs. 4A–C and 5**). Pathologic examination of the debrided tissue suggested inflamed synovial tissue with fragments of inflamed fibroadipose tissue with rare fragments of reactive bone. The patient went on to pain-free complete fusion of the tibial fibular joint and a pain-free ankle joint that improved with ambulation (see **Fig. 5**).

DISCUSSION

The most common indication for arthroscopy after TAR is soft tissue or bony impingement. Rates of residual pain owing to impingement range from 6% to 45% in the literature. [6,13] Residual pain after TAR can lead to decreased patient satisfaction and poorer outcomes. As a result, it is important to be able to properly manage this problem. Although rates of impingement may be high, the rate of patients requiring either open or arthroscopic debridement is relatively low. Kim and colleagues[9] studied 120 uncomplicated TARs with the Hintegra system with residual pain, of which only 7 patients (5.8%) went on to need arthroscopic debridement for impingement. Histology in these cases revealed "synovial hyperplasia with capillary ingrowth without the evidence of polyethylene debris."

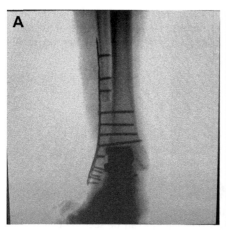
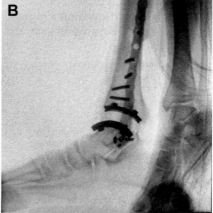

Fig. 2. (*A, B*) Intraoperative AP, medial, and lateral fluoroscopy views demonstrating a TAR with an attempted repair of the fibular nonunion and syndesmosis fusion.

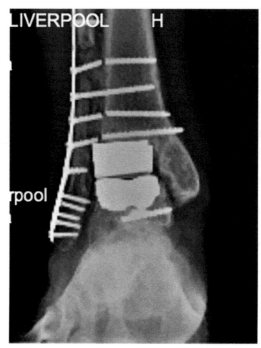

Fig. 3. AP radiograph demonstrating a nonunion of the tibial fibula syndesmosis fusion following the TAR procedure. The patient also presented with residual lateral gutter pain.

Outcomes after arthroscopic debridement are often excellent. Shirzad and colleagues[13] described their arthroscopic technique for managing impingement after TAR. They performed the technique on 11 patients, and all patients noted improvement in pain postoperatively. Richardson and colleagues[6] also reported their outcomes on 20 patients who underwent arthroscopic debridement. They found that 80% of patients initially reported improvement in symptoms, but ultimately 6 of the 20 patients required further revision.

The time at which patients present with residual pain as a result of impingement is variable and may depend on a multitude of factors, including the type of implant. A case series by Devos Bevernage and colleagues[10] reported an average time to

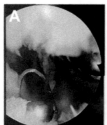
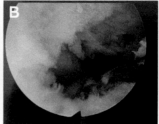
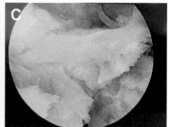

Fig. 4. Arthroscopic images of a TAR. (*A*) Notice the reflective talar component producing a mirrored image of the shaver. (*B*) The polyethylene spacer can be seen hidden by overgrowth of tissue and reflected by the talar component. (*C*) Fibrous tissue inside the joint contributing to impingement and pain.

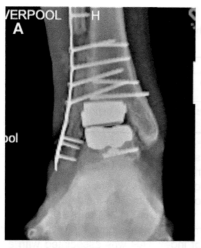
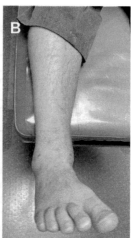
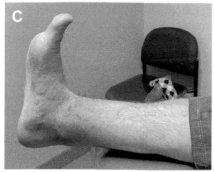
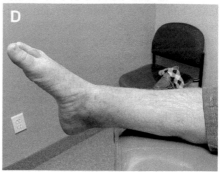

Fig. 5. (*A*) A postoperative AP ankle view. (*B*) A postoperative clinical view following the ankle arthroscopy procedure demonstrating the medial and lateral portal incision for the ankle arthroscopy and repair of the syndemotic non union. (*C*) A postoperative clinical view following the ankle arthroscopy demonstrating the range of motion and dorsiflexion following the surgery. Note the anterior medial portal. (*D*) A postoperative clinical view following the ankle arthroscopy demonstrating the plantarflexion following the surgery.

impingement after TAR was 38.2 months (range, 17–74 months). Three different three-component implants were used in this study (Ankle Evolution System, Mobility, and Hintegra). The investigators acknowledged that three-component systems may predispose a patient to gutter impingement owing to the freely movable polyethylene component.

However, impingement can also be seen with two-component fixed-bearing systems. One study by Gross and colleagues[15] did not find a significant difference between fixed- and mobile-bearing systems. However, they did report a significantly smaller rate of impingement with the Salto Talaris (2.7%) implant compared with the INBONE (8.5%) and STAR systems (10.0%; P = .002). They also found the mean time to debridement procedure after index TAR was an average of 38.7 months in STAR patients, 21.8 months in INBONE patients, and 10.5 months in Salto Talaris patients. These times to revision may be explained by the investigators' usage of implants over time with advances in implant design alongside a decreasing threshold to use arthroscopy as a tool for diagnosis and treatment of pain after TAR. Nevertheless,

Table 2	
Advantages and disadvantages of arthroscopy after total ankle replacement	
Advantages	**Disadvantages**
Less soft tissue trauma	Risk of neurovascular injury
Faster recovery and return to function	Risk of damage to implant components leading to third-party wear
Decreased risk of wound complications and deep infection	Inadequate debridement leading to continued pain and possible need for further surgery

the investigators' findings do not seem to suggest a predilection for impingement based on fixed- versus mobile-bearing implant designs.

Another study by Schuberth and colleagues[11,20] also reported the incidence of symptomatic impingement for various implants. The incidence was the lowest with the STAR (4%) and slightly higher for INBONE (11%) and Salto Talaris (12%). The mean time to debridement was 17 months. Interestingly, they also found that prophylactic gutter debridement at time of index TAR was associated with a significantly lower rate of symptomatic impingement postoperatively—2% in the prophylactic gutter debridement group versus 18% in the no gutter debridement group (*P*<.05). Therefore, these investigators highly recommend prophylactic gutter resection to prevent future impingement.

Although the outcomes of arthroscopic debridement for impingement after TAR are positive, it is also important to recognize the procedure's limitations alongside the potential benefits. In one comparative cohort study, 43 patients with anterior ankle spurring and no history of TAR were treated with either arthroscopy or open arthrotomy. The arthroscopy group fully recovered in 5 weeks, whereas the open group took 8 weeks to recover.[21] This faster recovery and return to function can be associated with less soft tissue trauma. Because of their location overlying the ankle joint, incision healing after an open arthrotomy may delay mobilization.

Although damage to the prosthesis can occur with both open and arthroscopic procedures, arthroscopic debridement and instrumentation alone can pose a risk to prosthesis components. Therefore, it may not be the first-choice procedure for inexperienced arthroscopists. Another limitation of arthroscopic debridement is the possibility of inadequate debridement. One study found that the rate of revision after arthroscopy was higher than after the open procedure; however, this did not meet statistical significance.[15] **Table 2** summarizes some of the advantages and disadvantages of arthroscopy after TAR.

COMPLICATIONS

As with any arthroscopic procedure, there is a risk of nerve and vascular injury, as well as deep infection. An additional complication that can occur when performing arthroscopy after TAR is iatrogenic damage to the prosthesis or poly. This can lead to body wear, which occurs when loose soft tissue or bone remains within the joint and further irritates the damaged area. The result of this damage is accelerated wear of the implant.[11] There is also a risk of malleolar fracture or excessive bony debridement with this procedure, which can result in destabilization of the implant components.[8,14]

SUMMARY

TARs continue to evolve with time, leading to improved survivorship and outcomes. Factors leading to impingement after TAR are multifactorial and often unclear;

however, it remains a common source of pain and cause of reoperation. Arthroscopy remains a beneficial and low-risk tool for exploration and treatment of symptomatic impingement.

CLINICS CARE POINTS

- Arthroscopic debridement for impingement after total ankle replacement is an alternative to open arthrotomy. Arthroscopy can allow for a quicker recovery and can reduce the risk of periprosthetic joint infection better than open arthrotomy.
- An open procedure is preferred in cases of severe heterotopic ossification or if other open procedures are required.
- The ankle should be placed in full dorsiflexion when establishing the arthroscopic portals to prevent damage to the prosthesis.
- A 2.7-mm arthroscope with a 70° camera may be useful to increase field of view and allow for access to tighter spaces to enable gutter debridement.
- Because of the highly reflective metallic components, a mirror image is visualized. Confusion can be avoided by orienting oneself through touch sensation.
- Multiple tools can be used for soft tissue and bone debridement. The use of a bipolar radiofrequency ablator is recommended for soft tissue and may be faster than using a shaver. The use of burrs, curettes, or an arthroscopic rongeur or punch is ideal for removal of ectopic bone.
- Adequate gutter debridement should allow arthroscopic visualization of the posterior tibial tendon medially, and the peroneal tendons laterally.
- Instruments should be shielded or directed away from the implant components at all times to reduce risk of harm. Iatrogenic damage to the prosthesis can result in third-body wear.

DISCLOSURE

Dr L. DiDomenico is a consultant to MTF, Zimmer Biomet, In2bones, Bone Support, Integra, and Paragon 28.

REFERENCES

1. Glazebrook MA, Arsenault K, Dunbar M. Evidence-based classification of complications in total ankle arthroplasty. Foot Ankle Int 2009;30(10):945–9.
2. Morash J, Walton DM, Glazebrook M. Ankle arthrodesis versus total ankle arthroplasty. Foot Ankle Clin 2017;22(2):251–66.
3. McKenna BJ, Cook J, Cook EA, et al. Total ankle arthroplasty survivorship: a meta-analysis. J Foot Ankle Surg 2020;59(5):1040–8.
4. Mann JA, Mann RA, Horton E. STAR (TM) ankle: long-term results. Foot Ankle Int 2011;32(5):473–84.
5. Gougoulias N, Khanna A, Maffulli N. How successful are current ankle replacements?: A systematic review of the literature. Clin Orthop Relat Res 2010; 468(1):199–208.
6. Richardson AB, Deorio JK, Parekh SG. Arthroscopic debridement: effective treatment for impingement after total ankle arthroplasty. Curr Rev Musculoskelet Med 2012;5(2):171–5.
7. Niek van Dijk C. Anterior and posterior ankle impingement. Foot Ankle Clin 2006; 11(3):663–83.

8. Lui TH, Roukis TS. Arthroscopic management of complications following total ankle replacement. Clin Podiatr Med Surg 2015;32(4):495–508.

9. Kim BS, Choi WJ, Kim J, et al. Residual pain due to soft-tissue impingement after uncomplicated total ankle replacement. Bone Joint Lett J 2013;95-B(3):378–83.

10. Devos Bevernage B, Deleu PA, Birch I, et al. Arthroscopic debridement after total ankle arthroplasty. Foot Ankle Int 2016;37(2):142–9.

11. Schuberth JM, Wood DA, Christensen JC. Gutter impingement in total ankle arthroplasty. Foot Ankle Spec 2016;9(2):145–58.

12. Chu AK, Brigido SA. "Addressing impingement issues after total ankle replacement." Hmpgloballearningnetwork.com, 2020, Available at: https://www.hmpgloballearningnetwork.com/site/podiatry/addressing-impingement-issues-after-total-ankle-replacement. Accessed May, 2020.

13. Shirzad K, Viens NA, DeOrio JK. Arthroscopic treatment of impingement after total ankle arthroplasty: technique tip. Foot Ankle Int 2011;32(7):727–9.

14. Lam HY, Lui TH. Arthroscopic decompression for medial ankle impingement after total ankle arthroplasty. Arthrosc Tech 2021;10(5):e1383–8.

15. Gross CE, Neumann JA, Godin JA, et al. Technique of arthroscopic treatment of impingement after total ankle arthroplasty. Arthrosc Tech 2016;5(2):e235–9.

16. Kurup HV, Taylor GR. Medial impingement after ankle replacement. Int Orthop 2008;32(2):243–6.

17. Gross CE, Adams SB, Easley M, et al. Surgical treatment of bony and soft-tissue impingement in total ankle arthroplasty. Foot Ankle Spec 2017;10(1):37–42.

18. Bemenderfer TB, Davis WH, Anderson RB, et al. Heterotopic ossification in total ankle arthroplasty: case series and systematic review. J Foot Ankle Surg 2020;59(4):716–21.

19. Lee KB, Cho YJ, Park JK, et al. Heterotopic ossification after primary total ankle arthroplasty. J Bone Joint Surg Am 2011;93:751–8.

20. Schuberth JM, Babu NS, Richey JM, et al. Gutter impingement after total ankle arthroplasty. Foot Ankle Int 2013;34(3):329–37.

21. Scranton PE Jr, McDermott JE. Anterior tibiotalar spurs: a comparison of open versus arthroscopic debridement. Foot Ankle 1992;13:125–9.

Arthroscopy of Foot and Ankle

Subtalar Joint Arthroscopy in Intra-articular Calcaneal Fractures

Shane Hollawell, DPM, FACFAS, Meagan Coleman, DPM, AACFAS*,
Sara Yancovitz, DPM, AACFAS

KEYWORDS

- Arthroscopy • Calcaneal fracture • Lateral extensile approach • Minimal invasive
- Sinus tarsi syndrome • Subtalar joint • Trauma

KEY POINTS

- Post-traumatic osteoarthritis of the subtalar joint is a devastating, yet common, sequela for acute intra-articular calcaneal fractures.
- Subtalar joint arthroscopy has been used in a variety of diagnostic and therapeutic procedures as a minimally invasive alternative to an open approach with extensive dissection.
- Subtalar arthroscopy with limited incision techniques is a valuable option that can assist in restoring articular congruency and can lead to improved long-term clinical outcomes.
- Subtalar joint arthroscopy can be used to relieve pain as well as potentially avoid subsequent arthrodesis or fusion in cases of intra-articular calcaneal fractures.

INTRODUCTION

The calcaneus is the most commonly fractured tarsal bone, with 60% to 75% of the fractures being displaced and intra-articular.[1] Many of these injuries are occupational and caused by an axial load from a fall. The injury is seen 2.4 times more frequently in men than in women.[2] Displaced intra-articular calcaneal fractures warrant surgical intervention as they risk painful malunions, advanced post-traumatic osteoarthritis and impingement-type symptoms if height and width of the calcaneus are compromised.[3,4] Most often, poor prognosis is associated with a step-off or malreduction in the posterior facet of the calcaneus.

The goals of surgical intervention for intra-articular calcaneal fractures include restoration of anatomic alignment of the height and width of the calcaneus, articular

Orthopaedic Institute Brielle Orthopedics, 2315 Route 34 South, Manasquan, NJ 08736, USA
* Corresponding author.
E-mail address: mcoleman@oiortho.com

Clin Podiatr Med Surg 40 (2023) 519–528
https://doi.org/10.1016/j.cpm.2023.03.004
0891-8422/23/© 2023 Elsevier Inc. All rights reserved.

podiatric.theclinics.com

congruency, and reduction of any rearfoot varus malalignment. The most challenging surgical objective is restoration of the articular surface within the subtalar joint. To restore the integrity of the articulation, the traditional surgical approach utilizes a lateral extensile incision for direct visualization, however, this incision poses a high risk for wound infection, dehiscence, and necrosis.[1] To mitigate these risks, minimally invasive techniques with subtalar joint arthroscopy complement intraoperative fluoroscopy to assess the quality of the articular reduction.[5]

Subtalar joint arthroscopy has been used in a variety of diagnostic and therapeutic procedures as an alternative to an open approach with extensive dissection. It was first described in the literature in the 1980s, and has been established to reliably evaluate the posterior facet of the talus and calcaneus.[6] Initially, arthroscopic assistance for calcaneus fractures was performed through a sinus tarsi approach in conjunction with an open procedure and has advanced as an adjunct for limited incision approaches. This approach was noted to be more reliable to restore the posterior facet than using solely intraoperative fluoroscopy with a traditional Broden's view.[5,6] The reason for the uncertainty is due to the unique shape of the subtalar joint which is concave in the transverse plane and convex in the sagittal plane. In addition, small, minute intra-articular incongruence can be overlooked on low-resolution fluoroscopic images, thus further challenging an accurate intraoperative assessment.

The gold standard to surgically treat intra-articular calcaneus fractures remains the lateral extensile approach; however, there is growing evidence that favors minimally invasive techniques (ie, sinus tarsi approach, closed reduction percutaneous pinning) to avoid risk for wound complications and skin breakdown.[7] In our clinical practice, we believe that the incorporation of subtalar arthroscopy with limited incision techniques is a valuable option that can assist in restoring articular congruence, decrease acute inflammation and can lead to improved long-term clinical outcomes.

Risks/Benefits/Indications/Contraindications

The main indications for subtalar arthroscopy include persistent sinus tarsi pain, subtalar joint impingement, chronic synovitis, osteochondral lesions, arthrodesis, coalition resection, removal of loose bodies, and os trigonum syndrome.[8] Advancements in technique have helped expand its indication to assist with reduction and fixation of intra-articular calcaneal fractures—which in many clinical scenarios warrant surgical intervention.

Absolute contraindications for subtalar arthroscopy in any clinical scenario include pre-existing advanced osteoarthritis or severe bone deformities that prevent access to the joint, in addition to, local soft tissue infection that pose risks for septic arthritis. Relative contraindications include poor skin quality or poor vascular status, and complex regional pain syndrome (CRPS).[8]

No major risks are associated with subtalar joint arthroscopy. Minor complications can occur, and are similar to any other arthroscopic procedure and include possible injury to nerves, bleeding, and infection. It has been noted that because there is a steep learning curve to the technique, a less experienced surgeon can dramatically increase the overall surgical time and potential post-operative complications.[9] In acute intra-articular calcaneal fractures, there is also a risk for the arthroscopic fluid introduction to exacerbate soft tissue swelling.

As subtalar joint arthroscopy can be used as an adjunct to limited incision treatment of calcaneal fractures, it lessens the risk of wound complications when compared to a lateral extensile calcaneal open reduction internal fixation (ORIF). Those complications include wound dehiscence, hematoma, and wound edge necrosis.[5] Furthermore, subtalar joint arthroscopy can also treat subtalar joint stiffness following an intra-articular calcaneal fracture which is the most prevalent complication following such injury.[2,3] Incorporating an arthroscopic release of arthrofibrosis following an ORIF of the fracture may provide dramatic pain relief, increased range of motion, and slow the onset of post-traumatic arthritis.

Literature Review

There are a limited number of reports that use subtalar arthroscopy in the reduction of calcaneal fractures. Nonetheless, their conclusions yield promising radiographic and clinical results. Schuberth and colleagues found excellent radiographic results in a retrospective analysis of 10 cases of minimally invasive, open reduction, and internal fixation for intra-articular fractures with arthroscopic assistance.[10] When comparing pre-operative to post-operative measurements, there were statistically significant improvements in posterior facet step-off, medial wall displacement, and Bohler's angle. Woon and colleagues found similar statistically significant improvements with Bohler's angle at 2 years post-operatively.[11] Good functional term results were found in a study by Rammelt and colleagues consisting of 18 patients with intra-articular calcaneal fractures who underwent arthroscopically assisted percutaneous fixation.[6] At 1-year post-op, these patients had an average American Orthopaedic Foot and Ankle Society (AOFAS) score of 94.1 points. In a study of 22 patients undergoing this surgical procedure, Woon and colleagues reported AOFAS scores of 84.2 ± 13.9 at 2 years post-operatively.[11]

There have been few complications reported in previous studies using a minimal invasive approach with the arthroscopic-assisted technique. There was a single case of a seroma and a separate case of portal site infection, both of which had resolved.[11,12] No other soft tissue complications were reported.[6,10,11] The low incidence of wound complications is much lower than the traditional approach which boasts complications of up to 24.9% using an extensile lateral approach to calcaneal fractures.[13] Furthermore, this technique has shown to be advantageous in populations with risk factors for healing due to its limited incision approach. Pastides and colleagues used a percutaneous arthroscopic approach to calcaneal osteosynthesis on 30 patients and only noted a single case of port site infection despite 58% identifying as smokers.[14]

Clinical Use of Subtalar Joint Arthroscopy

Intra-articular calcaneal fractures

Overall, intra-articular calcaneal fractures can be easily diagnosed. The patient typically presents after an acute high-energy traumatic event, such as a fall from a height or motor vehicle accident. Their symptoms often include pain, swelling, and the inability to bear weight. On physical exam, the hindfoot may be diffusely ecchymotic, appear to have a significant malaligned deformity when compared to their contralateral limb, and/or the surrounding skin can appear taut either at the lateral, posterior, or medial aspect of the hindfoot.[15] At the time of presentation, the clinician must also rule out compartment syndrome. Initial diagnosis of an intra-articular calcaneal fracture can be made using plain film radiographs. A complete view of the calcaneus, in addition to, a calcaneal axial view can aid in the diagnosis of an intra-articular calcaneal fracture. Positive radiographic findings include a "double density sign" seen on the lateral view, which can signify joint depression and subtalar joint incongruity.[15] On the calcaneal axial view, abnormalities in the sustentaculum tali, posterior facet, and hindfoot alignment can be determined. However, the gold standard in diagnosing an intra-articular calcaneal fracture is through advanced imaging of a computed tomography (CT) scan. A CT scan assists in quantifying comminution, articular facet displacement, and confirming any additional injury to surrounding osseous structures. Prior to surgical intervention, it is imperative that the patient has an adequate skin envelope absent of any concerns of soft tissue infection or unstable fracture blisters.

Other subtalar joint pathologies

Subtalar joint impingement, also known as sinus tarsi syndrome, is a condition that oftentimes can be misdiagnosed. Patients can complain of diffuse pain around the dorsal lateral hindfoot or direct focal pain within the sinus tarsi. Impingement pain can present either as sharp and acute, or dull and nonspecific, most often exacerbated by prolonged standing or ambulation. Additionally, the patient can present with a history of recurrent lateral ankle sprains or inflammatory arthritis.[16] The most common cause of this condition is an injury to the interosseous talo-calcaneal ligament. With the aid of MRI, advanced imaging may show significant amounts of synovitis with increased signaling within the sinus tarsi or evidence of direct injury at the interosseous talo-calcaneal ligament.[17] Furthermore, an MRI of the subtalar joint can appropriately identify fibrous coalitions, loose bodies, and even chondral defects. Subtalar joint arthroscopy can be a reasonable option when conservative management fails in addressing these subtalar joint pathologies.

Portal Placement

The major portals for subtalar joint arthroscopy consist of the middle, anterolateral, and posterolateral. The middle portal is placed directly over the sinus tarsi 1 cm anterior to the tip of the fibula, the anterolateral portal is placed 2 cm anterior and 1 cm distal to the tip of the fibula, and the posterolateral portal is at the tip of the fibula or parallel to the lateral Achilles border (**Figs. 1** and **2**). Typically, the majority of subtalar joint arthroscopy procedures can be performed using only the anterior and middle portals; however, the posterolateral portal provides good visualization of the posterior facet for critical reduction of calcaneus fractures. A thorough 13-point inspection should be performed to identify all surrounding anatomy (**Fig. 3**) and pathology within the subtalar joint, including synovitis and chondral defects (**Figs. 4** and **5**).

Case Study

This retrospective case study describes the surgical technique and functional outcomes in four patients (N = 4) who underwent open reduction internal fixation with concomitant subtalar joint arthroscopy due to an acute, closed, intra-articular, comminuted calcaneal fracture. It was concluded that concomitant subtalar joint arthroscopy is an advantageous and viable surgical procedure, that allows adequate visualization of the subtalar joint to ensure optimal anatomic reduction and decreases the risk of post-traumatic osteoarthritis, while keeping surgical risks and complication rates at a minimum.

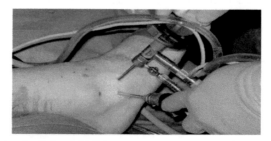

Fig. 1. Central and anterolateral portals.

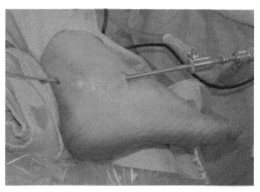

Fig. 2. Posterolateral portal.

A retrospective review of medical records, operative reports, physical therapy notes, and office visits was undertaken for patients with an acute closed, intra-articular, comminuted calcaneal fracture who underwent surgical intervention consisting of an open reduction internal fixation with concomitant subtalar joint arthroscopy. All surgeries were performed by a single board-certified surgeon (SMH). All chart reviews were assessed by an outside physician who was not the primary surgeon (MRC). Incomplete patient charts with missing data such as the operative report, missed appointments, and/or undocumented current post-operative milestones were excluded from this study. Patient demographics including age, gender, comorbidities, body mass index, and laterality of the injured extremity were recorded. Inclusion criteria included patients with the procedural code for an open reduction internal fixation of the calcaneus and subtalar joint arthroscopy over the age of 18 years.

All included patients had no previous injury to the lower extremities and were immediately consulted for their calcaneal fracture. Each patient had a minimum of 3 months of follow-up. The preoperative evaluation consisted of a thorough history and physical examination. Advanced imaging, consisting of a CT scan of the foot was ordered and reviewed before surgical intervention.

The number of days post-operatively that the patient was able to initiate protective weight bearing (PWB), initiate physical therapy (IPT), return to regular shoe gear (RSG), and return to full duty work status (RTW) were all recorded. The RTW status was defined as return to work full time with shifts greater than 8 hours with no modifications

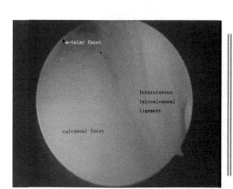
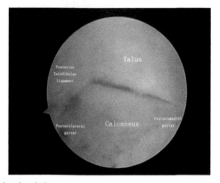

Fig. 3. Intraoperative 13-point inspection of subtalar joint anatomy.

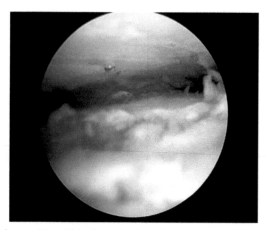

Fig. 4. Pathological synovitis within the subtalar joint.

or restrictions. The RSG was defined as running or tennis sneakers that were worn before surgical intervention. All patients included in this study were relatively active with minimal comorbidities. In addition, any complications or further treatment after the operative intervention were recorded.

Surgical Technique

From the time of initial consultation to the date of surgery, all patients were non-weight-bearing in a Jones compression posterior splint. Preoperative antibiotic was administered before surgical incision per typical protocol. The patient was placed on the operative table in a lateral decubitus position. Monitored anesthesia care with local infiltrate was used. All patients received a popliteal block before surgical incision. A proximal calf tourniquet was applied. A curved lateral extensile incision was made from the distal fibula to the distal calcaneal-cuboid joint. Blunt dissection was performed down to the level of the periosteum. A full-thickness flap was achieved and retracted with k-wires, using a no-touch technique, thereafter.

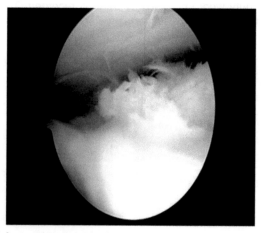

Fig. 5. Chondral defect within the subtalar joint.

The subtalar joint was grossly visualized. All fracture lines were dissected and identified. The lateral wall was removed to expose all articular fragments. A Steinmann pin was placed at the posterior calcaneus and a joystick maneuver was performed to reestablish appropriate height as well as to eliminate any varus positioning. Fluoroscopy was used to confirm the appropriate position of the calcaneal tuber. Subtalar joint arthroscopy was then performed after temporary k-wire fixation was placed subchondrally at the posterior facet and once the sustentaculum tali was temporarily fixated. A 30-degree, small joint scope was used. The articular surfaces of the subtalar joint were visualized to ensure complete anatomic alignment of all facets. Extensive joint debridement, in order to remove any aute hematoma or synovitis, was also performed at this time with a 1.9mm shaver. If the subtalar joint was noted to be misaligned or inadequately reduced, the k-wires were then backed out and repositioned. Once optimal reduction of the subtalar joint was completed, independent screws were placed from lateral to medial to support articular facets. The lateral wall was then reduced and a lateral calcaneal plate with corresponding locking and non-locking screws was placed through the plate.

Surgical incisions were then irrigated. A Jackson-Pratt size 10 round drain was placed in the lateral incision to prevent hematoma formation. The incision was then closed in a layer-by-layer fashion using 2-0 vicryl for deep closure, 4-0 monocryl for subcutaneous tissue, and 3-0 prolene for reapproximating the skin. Sterile dressing was applied to the incision followed by a well-padded posterior splint.

Patients were seen on a weekly basis for the first 3 weeks after surgical intervention, followed by every other week thereafter. Weekly appointments were deemed medically necessary for surgical dressing changes as well as to closely monitor for any signs of possible infection.

RESULTS

Four patients met the inclusion criteria. There were four feet ($N = 4$) which were evaluated. Of the four patients included in this study, 2 (50%) were male and two (50%) were female. The median age was 57.5 (range 52–63) years old. There were two (50%) calcaneal fractures that were included in the study that were injured due to a work-related incident. The median time follow-up was 681.5 (range 189–3,010) days. The median time between diagnosis of a closed, intra-articular, comminuted calcaneal fracture to surgical intervention was 15.5 (range 8–19) days (**Table 1**). Two of the four cases (50%) were due to a mechanical fall from a height greater than 10 feet from the ground. All patients were non-smokers, with minimal comorbidities. There was a single case (25%) who underwent primary subtalar joint arthrodesis, in addition to, open reduction internal fixation of the calcaneus and subtalar joint

Table 1 Patient demographics ($N = 4$)				
Patient	Age (years)	Gender	WRI (Y = yes, N = no)	MOI
1	53	M	Y	Fall from height, >10 ft
2	52	M	Y	Fall from height, >10 ft
3	63	F	N	Mistep off stairs
4	62	F	N	Mistep off stairs
Median	57.5			

Abbreviations: F, female; M, male; MOI, mechanism of injury; WRI, work-related injury.

arthroscopy. There was one (25%) case who underwent subsequent subtalar joint arthroscopy and did not have the arthroscopy performed at the time of open reduction internal fixation of the calcaneus. Subsequent arthroscopy was performed approximately 2 years after the initial open reduction internal fixation.

The median time post-operatively that the patient was able to initiate partial weight bearing was 58.5 (range 41–76) days. The median time post-operatively that the patient was about to IPT was 44.5 (range 41–76) days. The median time post-operatively that the patient was able to return to RSG was 93.5 (range 62–98) days. The median time post-operatively that the patient was able to return to normal activity was 130 (range 97–216) days. Finally, the median time that the patient was able to RTW status was 143.5 (range 97–216) days. The RTW status was defined as return to work full time with shifts greater than 8 hours with no modifications or restrictions (**Table 2**).

Complication rates were minimal, with no major complications encountered. One (25%) patient developed a hematoma to the lateral incision, which was manually expressed in the office. The patient was given oral antibiotics for 1 week for prophylactic measures and no further complications were documented. There were no reported cases of thromboembolic events, no surgical incision healing concerns, and/or wound dehiscence. In addition, there was no revision or reoperation surgery needed for any of the four cases.

DISCUSSION

Calcaneal fractures are devastating injuries that most often lead to post-traumatic osteoarthritis within the foot and ankle. Ensuring anatomical reduction of the calcaneus and all articular facets within the subtalar joint can help prevent early signs and symptoms of post-traumatic osteoarthritis. In addition, adequate articular reduction may allow a patient to return to normal activities of daily living and achieve pre-injury status without limitations such as joint stiffness, or pain. Subtalar joint arthroscopy can be used in conjunction with a minimal invasive approach to open reduction internal fixation of the calcaneus to visualize the posterior, middle, and anterior facets and to achieve an appropriate reduction of intra-articular fractures.

The use of subtalar joint arthroscopy to assist in the reduction of calcaneus fracture is a viable alternative to traditional approaches due to its overall low rate of post-operative complications. The most common complication is neuritis to branches of both the superficial peroneal nerve and the sural nerve due to portal proximity.[18] Establishing portals without injury and obtaining visualization within the subtalar joint may be

Table 2
Retrospective case study outcomes (N = 4)

Patient	Follow-up (Days)	Time Between Consultation-Surgery (days)	IPWB (Days)	IPT (Days)	RSG (Days)	RTA	RFD
1	3010	8	69	41	97	216	216
2	1159	19	76	76	98	98	113
3	189	15	41	41	90	162	174
4	204	16	48	48	62	97	97
Median	681.5	15.5	58.5	44.5	93.5	130	143.5

Abbreviations: IPT, initiate physical therapy; PWB, initiate partial weight bearing; RFD, return to full duty; RSG, return to regular shoe gear; RTA, return to normal activity.

challenging for inexperienced surgeons due to the small size of the joint.[19] Despite a steep learning curve to perform arthroscopic subtalar joint surgery, there continues to be technological advancements in instrumentation to ease the technical difficulty of the procedure.

This retrospective case study provides surgical outcomes of four patients who underwent open reduction internal fixation with concomitant subtalar joint arthroscopy to treat an acute closed intra-articular calcaneal fracture. Though small, this case study reinforces the favorable functional outcomes of previous studies, which is exemplified by the return to normal activity in normal shoe gear for all four cases at the 4-month post-operative mark (median = 130 days). In addition, this case study has a low complication rate compared to the current literature.

There are several limitations in our review of current literature for the use of arthroscopy in assisting reduction of calcaneal fractures. Most of the studies performed consisted of a small cohort size and had a short-term follow-up period. In addition, there is no consensus on which fracture pattern is best treated with the incorporation of subtalar joint arthroscopy. The range of severity using the Sanders classification varies between grades 2 and 3, and the results are not exclusive to either. We recommend that future studies should focus on increasing the number of cases included and extending the follow-up period to determine if patients develop post-traumatic arthritis, and if so, within what time frame.

SUMMARY

The use of subtalar arthroscopy and fluoroscopy in a minimal invasive approach to intra-articular calcaneal fractures provides dual modalities of visualization of the posterior facet for a more precise reduction. Current literature yields good functional and radiographic outcomes, less wound complications, and low incidence of post-traumatic arthritis with this technique than when utilizing an isolated lateral extensile incision of the calcaneus. As subtalar joint arthroscopy continues to grow in popularity and technological advancement, patients may benefit when surgeons incorporate this tool in conjunction with a minimally invasive technique for the treatment of intra-articular calcaneal fractures.

CLINICS CARE POINTS

- Subtalar joint arthroscopy used in assistance for reduction of intra-articular fractures can restore the articular congruence with a lower complication rate than traditional open reduction techniques.

- Computed tomography (CT) is the gold standard in diagnosing calcaneal fractures and aids in quantifying the extent of subtalar joint involvement.

- The majority of subtalar joint arthroscopy procedures can be performed using only the anterior and middle portals; however, the posterolateral portal provides good visualization of the posterior facet for critical reduction of intra-articular calcaneal fractures.

- The two most common causes of sinus tarsi syndrome are direct injury to the interosseous talo-calcaneal ligament and synovitis within the sinus tarsi.

- Concomitant subtalar joint arthroscopy can be critical in confirming the precise anatomical reduction of the articular facets in comminuted intra-articular calcaneal fractures.

- The most common complication of subtalar joint arthroscopy is neuritis of branches of the superficial peroneal nerve and/or sural nerve.

DISCLOSURE

There are no commercial and/or financial conflicts of interest, nor funding of any kind for all authors of this chapter.

REFERENCES

1. Sanders RW, Clare MP. Calcaneous fractures. In: Bucholz RW, Heckman JD, Court-Brown CM, et al, editors. Rockwood and green's fractures in adults. 7th edition. Philadelphia: Lippincott Williams & Wilkins; 2010. p. 2064.
2. Mitchell MJ, McKinley JC, Robinson CM. The epidemiology of calcaneal fractures. Foot 2009;19(4):197–200.
3. Rammelt S, Sangeorzan BJ, Swords MP. Calcaneal fractures - should we or should we not operate? Indian J Orthop 2018;52(3):220–30.
4. van Tetering EAA, Buckley RE. Functional outcome (SF-36) of patients with displaced calcaneal fractures compared to SF-36 normative data. Foot Ankle Int 2004;25(10):733–8.
5. Lui TH, Tong SC. Subtalar arthroscopy: when, why and how. World J Orthop 2015;6(1):56–61.
6. Rammelt S, Gavlik JM, Barthel S, et al. The value of subtalar arthroscopy in the management of intra-articular calcaneus fractures. Foot Ankle Int 2002;23(10):906–16.
7. Khazen G, Rassi CK. Sinus tarsi approach for calcaneal fractures: the new gold standard? Foot Ankle Clin 2020;25(4):667–81.
8. Muñoz G, Eckholt S. Subtalar arthroscopy: indications, technique and results. Foot Ankle Clin 2015;20(1):93–108.
9. Allegra PR, Rivera S, Desai SS, et al. Intra-articular calcaneus fractures: current concepts review. Foot Ankle Orthop 2020;5(3). https://doi.org/10.1177/2473011420927334. 2473011420927334.
10. Schuberth JM, Cobb MD, Talarico RH. Minimally invasive arthroscopic-assisted reduction with percutaneous fixation in the management of intra-articular calcaneal fractures: a review of 24 cases. J Foot Ankle Surg 2009;48(3):315–22.
11. Woon CY, Chong KW, Yeo W, et al. Subtalar arthroscopy and flurosocopy in percutaneous fixation of intra-articular calcaneal fractures: the best of both worlds. J Trauma 2011;71(4):917–25.
12. van Dijk CN, Scholten PE, Krips R. A 2-portal endoscopic approach for diagnosis and treatment of posterior ankle pathology. Arthroscopy 2000;16(8):871–6.
13. Nosewicz TL, Dingemans SA, Backes M, et al. A systematic review and meta-analysis of the sinus tarsi and extended lateral approach in the operative treatment of displaced intra-articular calcaneal fractures. Foot Ankle Surg 2019;25(5):580–8.
14. Pastides PS, Milnes L, Rosenfeld PF. Percutaneous arthroscopic calcaneal osteosynthesis: a minimally invasive technique for displaced intra-articular calcaneal fractures. J Foot Ankle Surg 2015;54:798–804.
15. Kim DH, Berkowitz MJ. Double density sign variant in fracture-dislocation of the calcaneus: clinical tip. Foot Ankle Int 2012;33(6):524–5.
16. Helgeson K. Examination and intervention for sinus tarsi syndrome. N Am J Sports Phys Ther 2009;4(1):29–37.
17. Pisani G, Pisani PC, Parino E. Sinus tarsi syndrome and subtalar joint instability. Clin Podiatr Med Surg 2005;22(1):63–77.
18. Donnenwerth MP, Roukis TS. The incidence of complications after posterior hindfoot endoscopy. Arthroscopy 2013;29(12):2049–54.
19. Donegan RJ. Improved anterior subtalar joint arthroscopy with a guide wire: a technique tip. Foot Ankle Int 2018;39(10):1219–22.

Arthroscopy for Traumatic Ankle Injuries

Glenn M. Weinraub, DPM[a],*, Arjun Vijayakumar, DPM[b]

KEYWORDS

- Ankle fracture • Arthroscopy • Traumatic ankle injury
- Open reduction internal fixation

KEY POINTS

- Anatomic reduction is the goal of treatment in the management of traumatic ankle injuries. A vast majority of the treatment revolves around open reduction and internal fixation.
- However, proposals for arthroscopic assisted approaches have been described to better assess intra-articular pathologies, with further benefits including less soft tissue exposure and prevention of trauma to local blood supply.
- The use of arthroscopy has been described in the treatment of medial malleolar fractures, syndesmotic injuries, pediatric ankle fractures, and pilon fractures.

INTRODUCTION

Ankle fractures are one of the most common types of injuries in adults that is associated with high rates of poor clinical outcomes.[1–3] Even after restoring the radiographic congruity of the ankle joint, clinically favorable outcomes are not always obtained.[4,5] Chronic pain in the joint after a fracture can be caused by a variety of intra-articular pathologies such as cartilaginous defects, loose bodies within the joint, and ligamentous damage, which can contribute to high rates of patient dissatisfaction.[6–8] Through standard open reduction and internal fixation (ORIF) of ankle fractures, these pathologies are unable to be properly diagnosed and subsequently addressed. For this reason, arthroscopy has been recommended by various authors in the management of acute ankle fractures to evaluate the joint for intra-articular injuries, provide a means for irrigation and debridement, and confirm the presence of anatomic reduction of joint surfaces and syndesmosis without the need for an arthrotomy to accomplish the same goals.[7,9–13] Additionally, arthroscopic assisted open reduction and internal fixation (AORIF), by way of a less invasive approach than traditional ORIF, can result in earlier mobilization, less postoperative pain, less prevalence of wound complications, and reduced complication or reoperation rates. Several studies have compared the use of AORIF to traditional ORIF of acute ankle fractures. In a study by Takao and

[a] Department of Orthopaedic Surgery, Kaiser Permanente, San Leandro, CA, USA; [b] Kaiser Permanente South Bay Consortium, Santa Clara, CA, USA
* Corresponding author. 2500 Merced Street, Building A, 4th Floor, San Leandro, CA 94577.
E-mail address: gmweinraub@gmail.com

Clin Podiatr Med Surg 40 (2023) 529–537
https://doi.org/10.1016/j.cpm.2022.12.003
0891-8422/23/© 2022 Elsevier Inc. All rights reserved.

colleagues,[14] 72 patients were randomly selected to either the AORIF or the ORIF group, and American Orthopedic Foot and Ankle Score (AOFAS) scores were measured in these groups after a mean duration of 40 months. The mean difference in AOFAS scores between the 2 groups showed a statistically significant difference, favoring the AORIF group. The authors of this study suggested that by visualizing the ankle joint through arthroscopy, diagnosis and subsequent treatment of intra-articular pathologies had a positive influence on clinical results after treatment of distal fibular fracture. This article will describe some specific instances where arthroscopic assisted treatment of acute ankle injuries has been utilized.

APPROACH

The ankle joint is well visualized using standard arthroscopic techniques that have been well established in prior literature.[15] The classic anteromedial and anterolateral portals are recommended, with establishment of the anteromedial portal performed first, followed by creation of the anterolateral portal. As is described in literature, damage to the superficial peroneal nerve with creation of the anterolateral port is frequently observed.[16] The identification of this nerve may be difficult in the setting of soft tissue swelling, secondary to acute trauma to the ankle joint. Nonetheless, accommodations can be made to decrease the risk of injury to this nerve by the use of a vertical skin incision, followed by blunt dissection to the level of the capsule and also by an inside-out technique, using the anteromedial portal to provide cutaneous transillumination to find the nerve.[17,18] Once the portals have been established, the primary author recommends the use of necessary equipment such as a dental pick, Kirschner wires, Weber large reduction clamps, and intraoperative fluoroscopy to assist with the evaluation and treatment of any intra-articular pathologies.

OSTEOCHONDRAL LESIONS OF THE TALUS

The incidence of osteochondral lesions of the talus has been reported in up to 69.4% of patients who had an acute ankle fracture. Furthermore, the frequency and severity of these lesions in the talar dome were found to be greater in patients with more severe ankle fracture patterns than in those with less severe ankle fracture patterns.[7,19] In a study by Stufkens and colleagues,[20] 147 patients had an arthroscopy performed to evaluate the extent of cartilage damage prior to surgical management of the ankle fracture, and results showed that initial cartilage damage of the anterior and lateral parts of the talar dome at the time of injury was found to significantly increase the risk of posttraumatic osteoarthritis. Although the rate of injury to talar cartilage after acute ankle fractures is high, the treatment of these chondral injuries at the time of injury and its effect on functional outcome scores remain undetermined. However, given the poor clinical outcomes of patients with ankle fractures and the high rates of osteochondral lesions associated with more severe ankle fractures, it is reasonable to assume that these intra-articular lesions may be contributing to the subpar results. To this effect, a study by Lantz and colleagues[21] demonstrated that patients who had simultaneous chondral lesions at the time of operative repair of acute ankle fractures had significantly poorer results than patients with ankle fractures without chondral lesions. In a study by Utsugi and colleagues,[22] higher rates of osteochondral defects were found in patients with poor functional outcomes at a mean duration of 12.4 months after ORIF of their ankle fractures. The evaluation of chondral lesions at the time of injury may lend important prognostic information in the management of these patients, as well as better patient outcomes postoperatively.

SYNDESMOTIC REDUCTION

Syndesmotic injury has been associated in up to 66% of acute ankle fractures. While the Lauge-Hansen classification system can predict syndesmotic injuries in rotational injuries, these injuries may not be evident in standard radiographic preoperative anteroposterior, mortise, and lateral views. A lack of proper diagnosis and treatment of a syndesmotic injury and even malreduction of a syndesmotic injury may be another reason why patients who have sustained ankle fractures have less favorable outcomes. Ogilvie and Reed showed significant syndesmotic disruption in patients who had persistent symptoms well after their ankle injury and who underwent arthroscopic debridement.[23] A way to fully diagnose syndesmotic injuries would be through ankle arthroscopy. In a study by Takao and colleagues,[24] ankle arthroscopy diagnosed 100% of cases with syndesmotic disruptions compared to 48% diagnosed by anteroposterior radiographs and 64% diagnosed by mortise radiographs. Furthermore, Lui and colleagues[25] found that 66% of their patients had arthroscopic evidence of syndesmotic diastasis, but only 30.2% had positive intraoperative stress radiographs. Patients were taken back to the operating room after 12 weeks for syndesmotic screw removal and for second-look arthroscopy. Ninety-one percent of these patients had regained stability of the syndesmosis, and Lui and colleagues suggested that ankle arthroscopy has the potential to assist in anatomic reduction of the syndesmosis.[25] However, ankle arthroscopy may also lead to overdiagnosis of syndesmotic instability in the absence of clinical indications of instability. As such, there is a potential for overtreatment of these injuries.[26]

LATENT SYNDESMOTIC INJURIES

In the setting of malreduction or even lack of reduction of the syndesmosis at the time of fixation, latent instability of the syndesmosis may be found. As a result, changes in joint contact areas and pressures have been described, leading to the progression of degenerative arthritis. These latent injuries were typically repaired using an open approach, resulting in acceptable outcomes.[27] One caveat of these open approaches, however, is the extent of soft tissue dissection, resulting in damage to anatomic structures that may lead to increased healing time and postoperative edema.[28,29] As discussed previously, arthroscopy can be a way to limit the harm to these structures while still accomplishing the goal of reducing and stabilizing the syndesmosis using a percutaneous fixation. As illustrated in **Figs. 1C** and **2**, the scope is placed through the anteromedial port, and the shaver is placed through the anterolateral port, in order to debride the syndesmosis of any scar tissue. The point of this process is to ensure the removal of tissue that would otherwise inhibit the reduction of the fibula into the tibial incisura (**Fig. 1**). In a study by Shuberth and colleagues,[30] 6 patients who had latent syndesmotic instability after a rotational ankle injury were followed up after a minimum of 2 years after arthroscopic assisted repair and percutaneous fixation to restore the ankle mortise. All these patients demonstrated significant improvement in pain and function at the final follow-up, as measured by the AOFAS scoring scale. The authors of this study were able to conclude that arthroscopic assisted treatment of latent syndesmotic instability was effective.

Pediatric Ankle Fractures

Another application of AORIF would be in pediatric ankle fractures. In adolescent patients, the asymmetric closure of the distal tibial physis, beginning centrally, progressing medially, and finishing anterolaterally, is believed to lead to transitional and triplane fractures.[31–33] Studies have shown that greater than 2 mm of intra-articular step-off

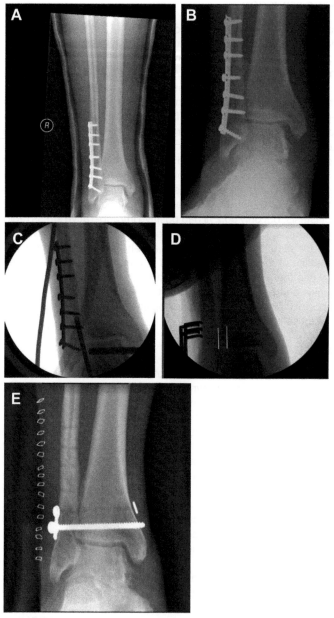

Fig. 1. (*A*) Postoperative radiograph after right ankle open reduction and internal fixation (ORIF). (*B*) Subsequent radiographs of the same ankle in the postoperative course demonstrating heterotopic ossification at the syndesmosis as well as increase in medial clear space. (*C*) Intraoperative fluoroscopy with a scope inserted into the anteromedial port and a shaver inserted into the anterolateral port, angled superiorly to facilitate debridement of syndesmotic debris. (*D*) Intraoperative external rotation stress test under fluoroscopy showing diastasis at the level of the syndesmosis after removal of prior hardware. (*E*) Postoperative films showing appropriate reduction of the syndesmosis and medial clear space with final fixation.

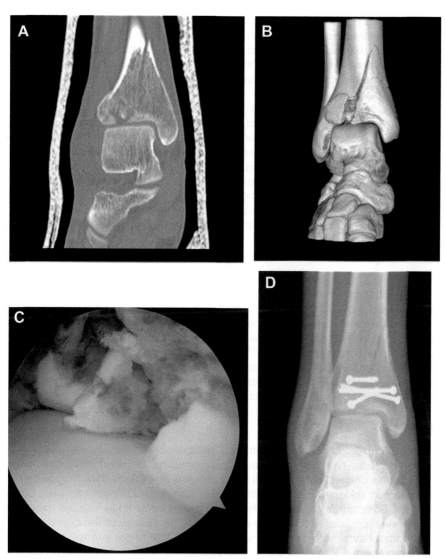

Fig. 2. (A) Computed tomography scan of a 43C-1-type pilon fracture. (B) Three-dimensional reconstruction images of the same injury depicting the anterior comminution. (C) Intraoperative fluoroscopic imaging showing the articular incongruity. (D) Final fixation using percutaneously placed cannulated screws.

should be treated with operative management.[31,34] In a study by Kling and colleagues,[35] a disturbance in growth was found in 1 patient out of 20 treated with ORIF, but growth disturbances were found in 5 out of 9 patients treated with casting. Percutaneous management of these fractures is frequently used, but arthroscopic assistance may be supplemented to ORIF to ensure reduction of the articular surface.

Salter-Harris III fractures account for roughly 25% of distal tibial fractures. Due to the nature of these injuries, there is often intra-articular incongruity. As such, there is a need for anatomic reduction of the articular surface to prevent the risk of joint incongruity and growth plate disturbance. A Tillaux fracture is a Salter-Harris III fracture of the anterolateral portion of the distal tibia. While growth arrest is not a concern in these types of fracture, the 2 mm of articular step-off still applies to prevent the development of posttraumatic arthritis. In a study by Jennings and colleagues,[36] 6 cases of arthroscopic assisted percutaneous fixation of intra-articular juvenile epiphyseal ankle fractures were shown to have comparable intermediate and long-term outcomes to ORIF of the same injuries.

Triplane ankle fractures are named as such due to the presence of fracture components in the sagittal, transverse, and coronal planes.[37] These fractures can appear similar to Salter-Harris III fractures on anteroposterior radiographs of the ankle and Salter-Harris II fractures on the lateral views. These injuries necessitate the use of computed tomography scans to properly determine the extent of articular step-off. As previously discussed, the indication for operative management is for displacement of greater than 2 mm or articular incongruity. The approach of arthroscopic assisted fixation of these fractures is mainly described in single case studies and case series[38,39] that have shown satisfactory results through the direct visualization of reductions.

PILON FRACTURES

Pilon fractures are caused by high-energy injuries associated with axial loading and possible rotational stress that extends into the articular surface of the tibial plafond. Literature has shown that the quality of anatomic reduction across the articular surface plays a large role in patient outcomes after ORIF of pilon fractures.[40,41] Arthroscopy can be a valuable asset at the time of fixation to determine the quality of articular reduction. Kralinger and colleagues[42] reported successful treatment of a closed distal tibial fracture through arthroscopic assisted reduction and fixation with percutaneous screws. They suggested that arthroscopy allows for more precise reconstruction of the tibial plafond through direct visualization.

LIMITATIONS

There are numerous risks and limitations associated with the use of AORIF. While some of these are typical of any arthroscopic procedure, the use of arthroscopy during acute trauma presents an additional tier of potential restrictions. The average complication rate in ankle arthroscopy is reported in a study by Zengerink and van Dijk as 10.3%.[43] Compartment syndrome has been described as a low-risk but dangerous complication associated with ankle arthroscopy. The etiology of the development of compartment syndrome has been assumed to be due to the extravasation of fluid that leaks into the lower extremity. One case of compartment syndrome has been described after the use of AORIF in the treatment of a Maisonneuve fracture.[44] While Ekman and Poehling[45] state that the risk of developing true compartment syndrome is low, it must still be taken into account as a potential consequence of AORIF. As described prior in this article, the risk of damage to the intermediate dorsal cutaneous nerve is present. While the use of ankle arthroscopy on its own has a steep learning curve, the concomitant use of ankle arthroscopy during ankle ORIF is more difficult still. With this added layer of complexity, one can expect the operative time for these procedures to increase. These factors must be taken into account when selecting patients as potential candidates for AORIF.

SUMMARY

Using ankle arthroscopy in conjunction to ORIF of traumatic ankle injuries can play an important role in the management of these injuries by way of treating intra-articular pathologies, leading to improved patient outcomes. While a majority of these injuries are not treated with concurrent arthroscopy, its addition may lead to more prognostic information to dictate the patient's course. This article has illustrated its use in managing malleolar fractures, syndesmotic injuries, pilon fractures, and pediatric ankle fractures. While additional studies may be needed to further support AORIF, it may prove to play a vital role in the future.

CLINICS CARE POINTS

- The use of arthroscopy during acute trauma presents additonal risks including compartment syndrome, damage to the intermediate dorsal cutaneous nerve, and increased operative time.

REFERENCES

1. Brown OL, Dirschl DR, Obremskey WT. Incidence of hardware-related pain and its effect on functional outcomes after open reduction and internal fixation of ankle fractures. J Orthop Trauma 2001;15(4):271–4.
2. Day GA, Swanson CE, Hulcombe BG. Operative treatment of ankle fractures: a minimum ten-year follow-up. Foot Ankle Int 2001;22:102–6.
3. Nilsson G, Nyberg P, Ekdahl C, Eneroth M. Performance after surgical treatment of patients with ankle fractures—14-month follow-up. Physiother Res Int 2003;8: 69–82.
4. Ferkel RD, Orwin JF. Arthroscopic treatment of acute ankle fractures and post-fracture defects. In: Ferkel RD, editor. Arthroscopic surgery. Philadelphia, PA: Lippincott Raven; 1996. p. 185–200.
5. Niek van Dijk C, Verhagen RAW, Tol JL. Arthroscopy for problems after ankle fracture. J Bone Joint Surg (Br) 1997;79-B:280–4.
6. Thordarson DB, Bains R, Shepherd LE. The role of ankle arthroscopy on the surgical management of ankle fractures. Foot Ankle Int 2001;22:123–5.
7. Leontaritis N, Hinojosa L, Panchbhavi VK. Arthroscopically detected intra-articular lesions associated with acute ankle fractures. J Bone Joint Surg Am 2009;91:333–9.
8. Ono A, Nishikawa S, Nagao A, Irie T, Sasaki M, Kouno T. Arthroscopically assisted treatment of ankle fractures: arthroscopic findings and surgical outcomes. Arthroscopy 2004;20:627–31.
9. Wood DA, Christensen JC, Schuberth JM. The use of arthroscopy in acute foot and ankle trauma: a review. Foot Ankle Spec 2014;7:495–504.
10. Takao M, Ochi M, Naito K, et al. Arthroscopic diagnosis of tibiofibular syndesmosis disruption. Arthroscopy 2001;17:836–43.
11. Salvi AE, Metelli GP, Bettinsoli R, Hacking SA. Arthroscopic- assisted fibular synthesis and syndesmotic stabilization of a complex unstable ankle injury. Arch Orthop Trauma Surg 2009;129:393–6.
12. Kong C, Kolla L, Wing K, Younger ASE. Arthroscopy assisted closed reduction and percutaneous nail fixation of unstable ankle fractures: description of a minimally invasive procedure. Arthrosc Tech 2014;3:e181–4.
13. Loren GJ, Ferkel RD. Arthroscopic assessment of occult intra-articular injury in acute ankle fractures. Arthroscopy 2002;18:412–21.

14. Takao M, Uchio Y, Naito K, Fukazawa I, Kakimaru T, Ochi M. Diagnosis and treatment of combined intraarticular disorders in acute distal fibular fractures. J Trauma 2004;57(6):1303–7.
15. Golanó P, Vega J, Pérez-Carro L, Götzens V. Ankle anatomy for the arthroscopist. Part I: the portals. Foot Ankle Clin 2006;11(2):253–73. PMID: 16798511.
16. Takao M, Ochi M, Shu N, et al. A case superficial peroneal nerve Inj during Ankle Arthrosc Arthrosc 2001;17:403–4.
17. Ferkel RD, Guhl JF, Heath DD. Neurol Complications Ankle Arthrosc Arthrosc 1996;12(35):200–8.
18. Barber FA, Britt BT, Ratliff HW, et al. Arthrosc Surg Ankle Orthop Rev 1988;17:446–51.
19. Hintermann B, Regazzoni P, Lampert C, Stutz G, Gachter A. Arthroscopic findings in acute fractures of the ankle. J Bone Joint Surg Br 2000;82:345–51.
20. Stufkens SA, Knupp M, Horisberger M, Lampert C, Hintermann B. Cartilage lesions and the development of osteoarthritis after internal fixation of ankle fractures: a prospective study. J Bone Joint Surg Am 2010;92:279–86.
21. Lantz BA, McAndrew M, Scioli M, Fitzrandolph RL. The effect of concomitant chondral injuries accompanying operatively reduced malleolar fractures. J Orthop Trauma 1991;5(2):125–8.
22. Utsugi K, Sakai H, Hiraoka H, Yashiki M, Mogi H. Intraarticular fibrous tissue formation following ankle fracture: the significance of arthroscopic debridement of fibrous tissue. Arthroscopy 2007;23:89–93.
23. Ogilvie-Harris DJ, Reed SC. Reed Disruption of the ankle syndesmosis: diagnosis and treatment by arthroscopic surgery. Arthroscopy 1994;10(5):561–8.
24. Takao M, Ochi M, Naito K, et al. Arthroscopic diagnosis of tibiofibular syndesmosis disruption. Arthroscopy 2001;17(8):836–43.
25. Lui TH, Ip KY, Chow HT. Comparison of radiologic and arthroscopic diagnoses of distal tibiofibular syndesmosis disruption in acute ankle fracture. Arthroscopy 2005;21:1370–4.
26. Robinson AHN, Sri-Ram K. Arthroscopic assessment of the syndesmosis following ankle fracture. Injury 2005;36:675–8.
27. Harper MC. Delayed reduction and stabilization of the tibiofibular syndesmosis. Foot Ankle Int 2001;22:15–8.
28. Cottom JM, Hyer CF, Philbin TM, Berlet GC. Transosseous fixation of the distal tibiofibular syndesmosis: comparison of an interosseous suture and endobutton to traditional screw fixation in 50 cases. J Foot Ankle Surg 2009;48(6):620–30.
29. Giebel GD, Meyer C, Koebke J, Giebel G. The arterial supply of the ankle joint and its importance for the operative fracture treatment. Surg Radiol Anat 1997;19:231–5.
30. Schuberth JM, Jennings MM, Lau AC. Arthroscopy-assisted repair of latent syndesmotic instability of the ankle. Arthroscopy 2008;24:868–74.
31. Herman MJ, MacEwen GD. Physeal fractures of the distal tibia and fibula. Curr Orthop 2003;17:56–62.
32. Rapariz JM, Ocete G, Gonzalez Herranz P, Lopez-Mondejar JA, Domenech J, Burgos J, Amaya S. Distal tibial triplane fractures: long-term follow-up. J Pediatr Orthop 1996;16:113–8.
33. von Laer L. Classification, diagnosis and treatment of transitional fracture of the distal part of the tibia. J Bone Joint Surg 1985;67A:687–98.
34. Spiegel PG, Cooperman DR, Laros GS. Epiphyseal fractures of the distal ends of the tibia and fibula. A retrospective study of two hundred and thirty-seven cases in children. J Bone Joint Surg Am 1978;60A:1046–50.

35. Kling TF Jr, Bright RW, Hensinger RN. Distal tibial physeal fractures in children that may require open reduction. J Bone Joint Surg Am 1984;66:647–57.
36. Jennings MM, Lagaay P, Schuberth JM. Arthroscopic assisted fixation of juvenile intra-articular epiphyseal ankle fractures. J Foot Ankle Surg 2007;46:376–86.
37. Kay RM, Matthys GA. Pediatric ankle fractures: evaluation and treatment. J Am Acad Orthop Surg 2001;9(4):268–78.
38. Whipple TL, Martin DR, McIntyre LF, et al. Arthroscopic treatment of triplane fractures of the ankle. Arthroscopy 1993;9:456–63.
39. Imade S, Takao M, Nishi H, et al. Arthroscopy-assisted reduction and percutaneous fixation for triplane fracture of the distal tibia. Arthroscopy 2004;20:123–8.
40. Chen SH, Wu PH, Lee YS. Long-term results of pilon fractures. Arch Orthop Trauma Surg 2007;127:55–60.
41. Jansen H, Fenwick A, Doht S, et al. Clinical outcome and changes in gait pattern after pilon fractures. Int Orthop 2013;37:51–8.
42. Kralinger F, Lutz M, Wambacher M, et al. Arthroscopically assisted reconstruction and percutaneous screw fixation of a Pilon tibial fracture. Arthroscopy 2003; 19:1–4.
43. Zengerink M, van Dijk CN. Complications in ankle arthroscopy. Knee Surg Sports Traumatol Arthrosc 2012;20:1420–31.
44. Imade S, Takao M, Miyamoto W, Nishi H, Uchio Y. Leg anterior compartment syndrome following ankle arthroscopy after Maisonneuve fracture. Arthroscopy 2009;25:215–8.
45. Ekman E, Poehling G. An experimental assessment of the risk of compartment syndrome during knee arthroscopy. Arthroscopy 2009;25:215–8.

Arthroscopic Treatment of the Septic Ankle

Jonathan C. Thompson, DPM, MHA[a],*, Ben M. Tonsager, DPM[b], Troy J. Boffeli, DPM[c]

KEYWORDS

- Arthroscopy • Septic arthritis • Pyarthrosis • Bacterial arthritis

KEY POINTS

- The septic ankle is a pathology that requires expeditious identification and management that requires an appropriate understanding of the diagnostic criteria as well as a high level of clinical suspicion.
- Arthroscopic management of the septic ankle provides an effective means to eradicate the infection and allows for stage-based guidance of treatment plan.
- The diagnosis and management of the septic ankle should ultimately rest on the clinical acumen of the experienced practitioner.

INTRODUCTION

Ankle joint sepsis is a relatively rare but potentially devastating pathologic process of the lower extremity. An incidence of approximately 7.8 cases per 100,000 individuals has been documented.[1] This pathology is more frequently encountered in the immunocompromised and intravenous drug user populations as well as in prosthetic joints but can less frequently be seen in those without clear comorbidities.[2] Morbidity associated with this diagnosis is approximately 10%, which illustrates its predilection for the critically ill or those with significant comorbidities.[1] Establishing the diagnosis of ankle joint sepsis is often challenging as it may present with concomitant pathologies and often lacks consistency in regard to classic clinical characteristics. Once a diagnosis has been established, prompt management is imperative to minimize the potential for long-term sequelae. The purpose of this article is to address the diagnosis and management of the septic ankle with a focus on arthroscopic treatment.

[a] Division of Orthopedics, Mayo Clinic Health System, 1400 Bellinger Street, Eau Claire, WI 54703, USA; [b] Foot & Ankle Surgical Residency Program, Regions Hospital/HealthPartners Institute, 640 Jackson Street, Saint Paul, MN 55101, USA; [c] Foot & Ankle Surgical Residency Program, Regions Hospital/HealthPartners Institute, TRIA Woodbury Orthopedic Center, Foot and Ankle Surgery, HealthPartners Medical Group, 640 Jackson Street, Saint Paul, MN 55101, USA
* Corresponding author.
E-mail address: thompson.jonathan@mayo.edu

Clin Podiatr Med Surg 40 (2023) 539–552
https://doi.org/10.1016/j.cpm.2023.02.007
0891-8422/23/© 2023 Elsevier Inc. All rights reserved.
podiatric.theclinics.com

CLINICAL PRESENTATION

While the clinical presentation of ankle sepsis is often variable, acute-onset monoarthritis exhibiting joint pain, edema, and stiffness raises clinical suspicion. However, such findings are nonspecific as a host of other differential diagnoses should be considered, including acute inflammatory arthropathies, gout, and similar pathologies (**Box 1**). Joint pain and history of joint edema have shown relatively high levels of sensitivity (85% and 78%, respectively). The presence of fever has proven to be inconsistent as a diagnostic factor with a sensitivity of 57%. Constitutional symptoms such as sweats and rigors are even less sensitive, exhibiting sensitivities of 27% and 19%, respectively.[3] Thus, due to the variability in presentation, such findings can contribute to the overall diagnostic picture, but the absence of 1 or several of these classic symptoms certainly cannot serve to rule out an infectious diagnosis. Patients with a history of diabetes mellitus, rheumatoid arthritis, immunosuppression, renal failure, human immunodeficiency virus, cirrhosis, late-stage cancer, intravenous drug use, history of joint surgery, or trauma have exhibited a higher risk for joint sepsis.[4–9] Conditions affecting the integrity of the skin or mucous membranes such as eczema, psoriasis, and ulcerations can serve as a portal for bacterial infection that can lead to joint sepsis via hematogenous inoculation[10] (**Box 2**). There should be a greater index of suspicion for patients in these populations. Additionally, immunosuppressed patients may exhibit a blunted clinical response in comparison to the typical patient population,[10] further contributing to the challenge of diagnosis in this high-risk group. Certainly, joint

---

Box 1
Differential diagnoses for acute monoarthritis

Infection

Rheumatoid arthritis

Gout

Pseudogout

Apatite-related arthropathy

Reactive arthritis

Systemic lupus erythematosus

Lyme arthritis

Sickle cell disease

Dialysis-related amyloidosis

Transient synovitis of the hip

Plant thorn synovitis

Metastatic carcinoma

Pigmented villonodular synovitis

Hemarthrosis

Neuropathic arthropathy

Osteoarthritis

Intra-articular injury

Adapted from Klippel et al. (Klippel JH, 2001) and Margaretten et al. (MArgaretten ME, 2007).

Box 2
Risk factors for joint sepsis
Diabetes mellitus
Rheumatoid arthritis
Gout and pseudogout
Immunosuppressive medications
End-stage renal disease
Systemic lupus erythematosus
Human immunodeficiency virus
Cirrhosis
Age >70
Late-stage cancer
Intravenous drug use
Recent surgery
Recent trauma
Skin diseases (psoriasis, eczema, ulcers)

sepsis can be seen in the healthy patient with no medical risk factors or underlying joint disease as this population constitutes up to 22% of all joint infections.[2]

DIAGNOSTIC CRITERIA

Establishing the diagnosis of ankle joint sepsis can be somewhat challenging due to variations in presentation and utility of diagnostic studies. Systemic laboratory results such as peripheral white blood cell (WBC) count, c-reactive protein, and erythrocyte sedimentation rate are generally variable and unreliable. While they may be elevated with ankle sepsis, they lack specificity and can also be elevated in the setting of inflammatory arthropathies.[4,11] Arthrocentesis of the ankle is necessary to obtain a sufficient diagnosis. Synovial fluid Gram staining is important in providing preliminary information before synovial culture results are available. It has been found to provide high specificity but is not overly sensitive, especially with certain pathogens. Gram stains have been shown to be positive in 71% of gram-positive cases,[12] 40% to 50% of gram-negative cases,[13–15] and 25% of gonococcal cases.[16] Additional investigations have found Gram staining to exhibit a false negative rate of 50.[17,18] Synovial cultures provide further diagnostic utility once available but have also only exhibited a sensitivity of 82%.[19]

White-blood cell counts of synovial fluid provide additional diagnostic clarity and should be performed when there is sufficient aspirate to do so. No specific threshold is diagnostic for joint sepsis; however, the likelihood increases with higher synovial WBC values. Synovial WBC values greater than 50,000 cells/mm^3 are five times more likely to be consistent with SA while values greater than 100,000 cells/mm^3 are considered very strong predictors for a positive diagnosis.[6] However, a lower cell count certainly does not definitively rule out a septic joint. Li and Henderson found that one-third of septic joint patients had a synovial WBC of less than 50,000 cells/mm^3.[11] Cell counts as low as 6000 cells/mm^3 have been reported.[6] Patients exhibiting these abnormally low synovial WBC cell counts typically tend to be critically ill with organ failure and immunosuppression.[9] Thus, a high level of scrutiny is warranted in these patient populations as there is greater potential for deviation from the typical presentation. Additionally, the percentage of polymorphonuclear cells in joint aspirate can provide additional diagnostic utility as a value of at least 90% has been strongly associated with SA.[19–21] Synovial glucose and lactate values have also been shown to be effective diagnostic markers.[22]

Certainly, acute gout is a common differential that should be considered in the adult patient with acute monoarthritis. Thus, a joint fluid analysis should include synovial crystal evaluation. However, aspirate that is positive for crystalline arthropathy does not rule out a concomitant infectious etiology as the incidence of both is estimated at 1.5%.[8] Synovial WBC counts are often elevated with acute inflammatory arthropathies as are systemic blood WBC and inflammatory markers, further clouding the specificity of these studies. In the setting of a positive synovial crystal result, it is reasonable to initiate the appropriate treatment while continuing to await culture results to rule out a concomitant infectious etiology.

Blood cultures are also recommended as part of the workup for ankle sepsis. Bacteremia has been seen in at least one-third of SA patients as a hematogenous etiology is common. Twenty percent of septic joint cases have negative cultures,[23] so up to 14% of septic joint patients rely on a bacteremia diagnosis to establish a bacterial etiology.[24,25]

The diagnosis of ankle joint sepsis can at times be rather elusive. There are a host of factors that can confound a septic joint diagnosis. The Newman criteria provide general diagnostic guidelines for arriving at a septic joint diagnosis: positive synovial fluid culture, positive blood cultures with concomant clinical features of a septic joint with synovial cultures being negative, or negative cultures but clinical evidence of infection with purulent joint fluid (synovial fluid WBC count >100 kg/mL) without evidence of synovial fluid crystals.[26] This can provide the practitioner with general diagnostic assistance but cannot be used as an absolute guide. The results of synovial labs should be considered in conjunction with clinical history and comorbidities in order to establish an index of suspicion for a positive diagnosis. It has been asserted that while various diagnostic criteria assist in obtaining a more complete clinical assessment, there is no substitute for the suspicion of an experienced practitioner in establishing the diagnosis of joint sepsis.[27]

Diagnostic Aspiration Technique

Diagnostic aspiration of the ankle should be performed when clinical suspicion for joint sepsis exists. This can be performed through a standard anteromedial ankle approach, immediately medial to the tibialis anterior tendon and lateral to the greater saphenous vein (**Fig. 1**). These landmarks can be best palpated when the patient is holding their foot in a ninety-degree position against slight resistance to accentuate the firing of the tibialis anterior tendon. Our preference is to then mark the injection location with an indelible marker prior to prepping the injection site with betadine or chlorhexidine. This prevents the need to repalpate the landmarks with sterile gloves after prepping and obviates the need for sterile gloves. Infiltration of local anesthetic as a field block proximal to the aspiration site can be performed as needed at the discretion of the clinician. A 16- to 18-gauge needle is attached to a Luer-lock syringe of at least 10 mL in order to provide sufficient suction for aspiration. The foot is held in a neutral position during aspiration to minimize potential for iatrogenic chondral injury during aspiration (**Fig. 2**). In the septic joint, extensive intra-articular synovitis is often encountered and may impede aspiration, so redirection of the needle multiple times may be necessary to obtain an appropriate amount of aspirate. After the aspirate is

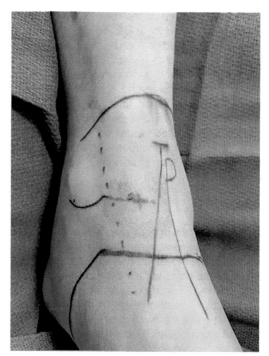

Fig. 1. Landmarks for an anteromedial ankle portal approach for joint aspiration.

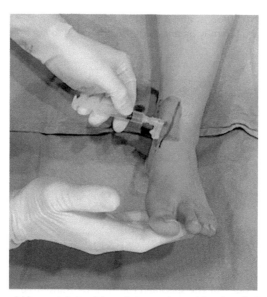

Fig. 2. The foot should be maintained in a right-angle position in relation to the lower leg during aspiration to minimize the potential for iatrogenic chondral injury.

obtained, a sterile twist cap is placed on the Luer-lock syringe prior to being placed in a specimen bag and transported to the microbiology laboratory (**Fig. 3**). It is not uncommon that the volume of joint fluid that can be aspirated may be insufficient to complete all the necessary tests, so prioritizing which labs are performed first is important. The authors practice in multispecialty health system settings and will routinely contact the laboratory to confirm the order of testing. First priority should be given to aerobic and anaerobic cultures and Gram staining followed by cell count and crystal analysis. While certain specimens may be diluted in the laboratory in the event of low aspirate volume, the portion of specimen used for cell count should not be diluted as this will confound the results. The patient is instructed to maintain non per os status while awaiting the results of the initial Gram staining and cell count in the event a surgical intervention may be needed.

TREATMENT

In the event of a positive diagnosis or high suspicion of ankle sepsis, immediate treatment should be initiated. The general consensus for treatment includes pursuing antibiotic therapy with prompt removal of purulent material from the joint space.[28] Guidelines have asserted the need to "aspirate to dryness as often as required."[28] However, discrepancy remains in regard to whether arthrocentesis versus surgical lavage is more appropriate. A meta-analysis from 1986 evaluated research over a 25-year period comparing outcomes with aspiration versus surgical arthroscopic or open debridement of all septic joints. These results yielded a significant difference in good outcomes for joint aspiration over surgery (73.7% vs 55.9%, $P < 0.05$).[29] Weston and Jones performed a subsequent retrospective review exhibiting better functional outcomes with arthrocentesis than with surgery although mortality was found to be higher in the arthrocentesis cohort.[2] Two more recent retrospective studies found no significant difference in the outcomes between the aspiration and surgical groups.[30,31] A 2019 investigation by Harada and McConnell reported on a 10-year retrospective review showing no statistically significant difference between outcomes of the two groups at 12 months postoperatively.[32] They concluded that closed-needle aspiration may be an adequate approach to the treatment of native joint

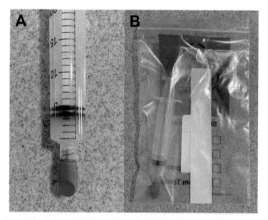

Fig. 3. (A) Joint aspirate from a patient with a septic ankle diagnosis. A sterile cap is secured on the Luer-lock syringe. (B) The specimen can then be transferred to the laboratory in a specimen bag where staff can transfer the aspirate to the appropriate tubes for the ordered tests.

infections.[32] However, such comparative studies include all joints, and typically septic ankle cases constitute a small subset of these cohorts. It is not clear from the available literature to what extent outcomes can be extrapolated between joints. Potential for selection bias in such studies should also be considered, as it may be surmised that clinically more severe infections might be more apt to be surgically addressed. Dissimilarly, severely ill patients may not be ideal surgical candidates and more likely to undergo arthrocentesis. Such factors confound clear recommendations between aspiration and surgical management.

Septic arthritis is generally considered a medical emergency requiring emergent intervention. This has been due to the potential for septicemia and adjacent osteomyelitis as well as to reduce the potential for cartilage injury.[3,17,27,33–39] However, 1 retrospective review of 204 cases spanning 18 years found patients had similar outcomes whether treated within six hours, between six to twenty-four hours, or greater than twenty-four hours and asserted that emergent surgical intervention may not be necessary in the absence of clinical sepsis.[40] The standard recommendation continues to be for prompt intervention once a positive diagnosis or high suspicion for it is reached.

Antibiotic Treatment

Given that there can be difficulty in establishing a septic ankle diagnosis, there should be a low threshold for initiating parenteral antibiotic therapy if suspicion is high. The most common causative organisms are *Staphylococcus aureus* followed by *Steptococcus*.[41] Gram-negative infections are less common but seen with greater frequency in critically ill patients, the elderly, intravenous drug users, or immunocompromised patients. Broad-spectrum antibiotics should be initiated early and tailored to culture sensitivities as available. Given the relatively high frequency of methicillin-resistant *Staphylococcus aureus*, empiric coverage with vancomycin or similar antibiotic should be initiated. For those patients considered at greater risk of gram-negative infection, the appropriate antibiotic such as cefepime should be considered.[10] Multidisciplinary management of the septic ankle patient with infectious diseases is appropriate when feasible.

Medical Treatment

Joint arthrocentesis in conjunction with parenteral antibiotics can be an acceptable means of addressing ankle joint sepsis. General recommendations in regard to technique and frequency are largely not based on high-level research nor are they specific to the ankle. General orthopedic recommendations include daily arthrocentesis that should be repeated until effusions resolve and cultures are negative. With this approach, surgical intervention is indicated if there is failure to respond after five to seven days of daily arthrocentesis with parenteral antibiotics or if there is soft tissue extension of infection.[42,43] Arthrocentesis guidelines that have been described in the wrist consist of serial aspirations on a daily basis until wrist improvement, no fluid is removed, or after two to three days of no clinical improvement at which time operative intervention may be necessary.[9] Both infiltrating the joint with sterile saline during aspiration and joint catheters have also been described, but aspirating the joint to dryness is the more commonly recommended approach.[9] Given that arthrocentesis has been shown to be an effective initial treatment for joint sepsis, it can be surmised that this could be an appropriate treatment option for an acutely diagnosed septic ankle if emergent referral is not available to a surgeon adept in ankle arthroscopy. Alternately, this may be a reasonable initial approach if a clear diagnosis has not yet been achieved but clinical suspicion for SA is high.

Surgical Treatment

Surgical arthroscopy or arthrotomy is indicated in the septic ankle patient as an initial intervention or after failing a serial aspiration approach. Arthroscopy is the authors' preferred approach in the majority of cases as it not only serves to decompress the joint and evacuate the infectious nidus but also allows for targeted lavage in a manner perhaps superior to an open approach. More precise debridement of the intra-articular space is often feasible with this approach. Additionally, arthroscopy is typically minimally disruptive to the surrounding edematous skin and provides the ability to appropriately stage the joint, which serves to direct treatment. However, at times, arthrotomy may be necessary in the late-stage septic joint or if extension into the surrounding soft tissues or bone has occurred.

Prompt surgical arthroscopy is pursued after a diagnosis of pyarthrosis is made or if clinical suspicion is high. Surgery is performed under general anesthesia in the supine position. Joint distraction is not used as it is generally not necessary to sufficiently access the joint and avoids unwarranted injury to the surrounding edematous soft tissue envelope. Standard anteromedial and anterolateral ankle portals are used as outlined by Ferkel.[44] The ankle joint is insufflated with sterile saline via the anteromedial approach similar to the technique used for standard elective ankle arthroscopy. The anteromedial portal is then established immediately medial to the tibialis anterior tendon and lateral to the greater saphenous vein. Either a 2.7-mm or 4.0-mm arthroscope is used per surgeon preference although the larger scope may be more amenable to high-volume lavage of the joint. The anterolateral portal is then established with the assistance of transillumination. This approach can assist with establishing the second portal at the appropriate level while also providing visualization of the lateral border of the extensor digitorum longus tendons. Care should also be taken to avoid the intermediate dorsal cutaneous nerve when establishing this portal. The nerve can at times be visualized clinically in the typical patient by slightly plantarflexing and inverting the foot. It is unlikely this technique would be beneficial in the edematous tissues of an SA patient, so transillumination can at times provide visualization of the nerve. Alternately, inspection of the nerve location on the unaffected limb may inform the surgeon of its location on the operative extremity.

Once both portals are established, obtaining predebridement intra-articular specimens is prudent. While there are no firm criteria for specimen procurement, our preference is to obtain at least 1 deep aerobic and anerobic culture specimen as well as a soft-tissue pathology specimen of hypertrophic synovitis. If the patient has not yet been started on intravenous antibiotics, they should be held until these cultures are obtained intraoperatively. It is not uncommon in the septic ankle that initial inspection of the joint may yield extensive synovitis to the point where it is difficult to visualize the articular surface or establish clear landmarks. Careful initial blind debridement may be necessary before the joint surface can be visualized, with care being taken to avoid the articular surface or surrounding neurovascular structures. Intraoperative fluoroscopy can be beneficial in guiding correct portal placement when visualization is poor. When irrigating the joint, the authors use unimpregnated lactated Ringer's (LR) solution, and while clear guidelines on appropriate fluid volume are lacking, we generally recommend a minimum of 9 L of fluid, with more being indicated based on the extent of involvement. Isolated antibiotic-impregnated LR or a combination of both impregnated and unimpregnated LR has also been described.[45] Kirchhoff and Braunstein describe using 10 to 15 L of sterile fluid.[46] Mankovecky and Roukis used a range of 9 to 60 L of fluid in a case series of eight septic ankles, basing the amount of fluid needed on the stage of infection and extent of debridement required.[45]

Once feasible, a thorough twenty-one-point inspection of the joint is performed.[44] This allows for appropriate staging of the septic joint per the criteria put forth by Gäechter,[47] who established a stage-based protocol on the extent and frequency of debridement that is typically necessary. This approach was subsequently reported on in the general septic joint literature by Stutz and Kuster followed by Vispo-Seara and Barthel before being described in the ankle by Boffeli and Thompson.[34,48,49] A stage I septic joint exhibits synovitis and turbid fluid with possible petechiae. Generally, single arthroscopic irrigation with minimal debridement is sufficient at this stage. Stage II SA displays fibrin deposits, purulence, and inflammation and can often be sufficiently addressed with irrigation and debridement with local synovectomy and fibrinectomy. It is likely that repeat surgical debridement would be necessary. Stage III exhibits synovial thickening and formation of multiple pouches caused by adhesions. Multiple irrigation and debridement procedures including adhesion resection and partial-to-subtotal synovectomy can be anticipated at stage. End-stage septic joints exhibit aggressive synovitis, radiographic changes, and subchondral erosions and may be more likely in situations of delayed diagnosis. Advanced imaging such as MRI should be considered in these patients to evaluate for involvement of adjacent osseous structures and possible extension into the soft tissues. These stage IV findings often warrant consideration of ankle arthrotomy with multiple irrigation and debridement procedures, removal of loose fragments, and curettage of erosions or cysts. If there appears to be osseous involvement based on preoperative imaging or intraoperative findings, bone cultures and pathology should be obtained per routine techniques. The septic joint stage–based protocol can be seen in **Table 1**, and an example of intraoperative arthroscopic appearance is displayed in **Fig. 4**. While this stage-based treatment protocol provides general guidance on anticipated management, it should not be applied in isolation as it is prudent to consider overall clinical trajectory in determining the need for future debridement. The arthroscopy portals are generally not sutured to allow the joint and surrounding tissues to drain unimpeded.

Table 1
Stage-based treatment protocol for the septic ankle joint

Stage	Intraoperative Findings	Surgical Treatment
I	Synovitis, turbid fluid, possible petechiae	Single arthroscopic irrigation with minimal debridement
II	Fibrin depositions, purulence, inflammation	Irrigation and debridement with local synovectomy and fibrinectomy, likely to repeat surgery
III	Synovial thickening, formation of multiple pouches caused by adhesions	Multiple irrigation and debridement surgeries, with adhesion resection and partial to subtotal synovectomy
IV	Aggressive synovitis, radiographic changes, subchondral erosions	Consider arthrotomy with multiple irrigations and debridements, removal of loose fragments, and curettage of erosion or cysts

Adapted from Boffeli et al with permission (Boffeli TJ, 2015).

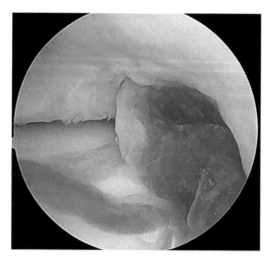

Fig. 4. Intraoperative arthroscopy images display an example of stage II ankle sepsis.

Guidelines for returning to the operating room for repeat irrigation and debridement are largely expert opinion-based and lack sufficient high-level support. Takahashi and Kajita recommended considering the following factors to determine the need for repeat surgery in elbow SA: (1) clinical presentation of fevers, persistent pain, and limitation of motion; (2) abnormal laboratory values like the persistent elevation of WBC

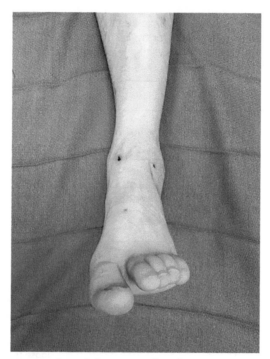

Fig. 5. The arthroscopy portals are left open to allow for postoperative exudate extravasation. Local wound care generally with a nonadherent dressing is advocated until wound healing is achieved.

count and c-reactive protein level; (3) no decrease in postoperative wound drain output volume.[50] While drain placement has not regularly been described in septic ankle management, these remaining factors warrant consideration in determining when repeat surgical intervention is necessary. Dave and colleagues found in knee SA the number of surgical interventions and likelihood of treatment being unsuccessful significantly decreased when time to intervention was minimized, so cases with a delayed diagnosis may be more likely to require a repeat surgery.[51] We consider persistently elevated infectious and inflammatory markers as well as trajectory of ankle pain and mobility in the days after the index surgery, generally repeating surgical debridement every two to three days as indicated based on these findings.

Our postoperative protocol consists of boot immobilization and non-weight-bearing for two to four weeks postoperatively prior to transitioning into an ankle brace with slow progression of activity as tolerated. Regular early ankle range of motion is emphasized to minimize the potential for functional deficits. Wound care measures are pursued at the open portal sites until healing is achieved (**Fig. 5**). Guidelines for duration of antibiotic therapy are sparse and generally range from three to six weeks of intravenous antibiotics in the adult SA patient.[10] Coordination with an infectious diseases or internal medicine specialist is important throughout the period of antibiotic administration. It is prudent to follow laboratory values until they normalize and obtain serial radiographs at two to three months postoperatively to rule out signs of latent infection.

SUMMARY

The septic ankle is a pathology that requires expeditious identification and management. Diagnosis of the pathology not only requires an appropriate understanding of the diagnostic criteria but also relies heavily on clinical suspicion. If certain classic diagnostic criteria are not met but index of suspicion for SA remains high, it should not be ruled out as a differential diagnosis. Prompt intervention is necessary to minimize the potential for suboptimal outcomes. Arthroscopic management in most cases provides an effective means to eradicate the infection. It allows for stage-based guidance in determining the extent and frequency of debridement that may be required. Reliance on arthroscopic stage-based treatment should not be absolute as there is potential for deviation and atypical presentation. The diagnosis and management of this at-times-challenging pathology should ultimately rest on the clinical acumen of the experienced practitioner.

CLINICS CARE POINTS

Pearls & Pitfalls from Arthroscopic Treatment of the Septic Ankle

Pearls
- Arthroscopic staging of the septic ankle can assist in determining the extent and frequency of surgical debridement.
- Palpation of typical arthroscopic landmarks may be difficult due to edema; intraoperative fluoroscopy can be helpful in confirming appropriate portal placement.
- Arthroscopy portals can be left open to allow for drainage with healing via secondary intention similar to extra-articular infection principles.
- Consider advanced imaging to rule out extra-articular infectious nidus if response to treatment is insufficient.

Pitfalls
- Diagnostic aspiration through cellulitic tissue has joint inoculation potential and should be avoided when possible.

- Aspirates that are positive for crystalline arthropathy do not rule out the possibility of a concomitant septic ankle joint.
- Laboratory values and clinical presentation may be underwhelming in the immunocompromised patient and can obscure the diagnostic criteria in this patient population.
- Delayed diagnosis of the septic ankle significantly increases morbidity, so a low index of suspicion for treatment is appropriate.

DISCLOSURE

T.J. Boffeli: Ownership in Surgical Design Innovations and investor in ExoToe, LLC.

REFERENCES

1. Kaandorp CJ, Van Schaardenburg D, Krijnen P, et al. Risk factors for septic arthritis in patients with joint disease. A prospective study. Arthritis Rheum 1995;38:1819–25.
2. Weston VC, Jones AC. Clinical features and outcome of septic arthritis in a single UK Health District. Ann Rheum Dis 1999;58:214–9.
3. Margaretten ME, Kohlwes J. Does this adult patient have septic arthritis? J Am Med Assoc 2007;297:1478–88.
4. Skeete K, Hess EP. Epidemiology of suspected wrist joint infection versus inflammation. J Hand Surg 2011;36:469–74.
5. Goldenberg DL, Brandt KD. Treatment of septic arthritis: comparison of needle aspiration and surgery as initial modes of joint drainage. Arthritis Rheum 1975; 18:83–90.
6. Yu KH, Luo SF. Concomitant septic and gouty arthritis-an analysis of 30 cases. Rheumatology 2003;42:1062–6.
7. Sammer DM, Shin AY. Comparison of arthroscopic and open treatment of septic arthritis of the wrist. J Bone Joint Surg Am 2009;91:1387–93.
8. Shah K, Spear J. Does the presence of crystal arthritis rule out septic arthritis? J Emerg Med 2007;32:23–6.
9. Claiborne JR, Branch LG. An algorithmic approach to the suspected septic wrist. Hand Surg 2017;78(6):659–62.
10. Ross JJ. Septic arthritis of native joints. Infect Dis Clin 2017;31:203–18.
11. Li SF, Henderson J. Laboratory tests in adults with monoarticular arthritis: can they rule out a septic joint. Acad Emerg Med 2004;11:276–80.
12. Goldenberg DL, Cohen AS. Acute infectious arthritis. Am J Med 1976;60:369–77.
13. Goldenberg DL, Brandt KD. Acute arthritis due to gram-negative bacilli: a clinical characterization. Medicine (Baltim) 1974;53:197–208.
14. Bayer AS, Chow AW. Gram-negative bacillary septic arthritis: clinical, radiographic, therapeutic, and prognostic features. Semin Arthritis Rheum 1977;7: 123–32.
15. Newman ED, Davis DE. Septic arthritis due to gram negative bacilli: older patients with good outcome. J Rheumatol 1988;15:659–62.
16. Goldenberg DL, Reed JI. Bacterial arthritis. N Engl J Med 1985;312:764–71.
17. Mathews CJ, Kingsley G. Management of septic arthritis: a systematic review. Postgrad Med 2008;84:265–70.
18. McGillicuddy DC, Shah KH. How sensitive is the synovial fluid white blood cell count in diagnosing septic arthritis. Am J Emerg Med 2007;25:749–52.

19. Krey PR, Bailen DA. Synovial fluid leukocytosis: a study of extremes. Am J Med 1979;67:436–42.
20. Shmerling RH, Delbanco TL. Synovial fluid tests: what should be ordered? JAMA 1990;264:1009–14.
21. Kortekangas P, Aro HT. Synovial fluid leukocytosis in bacterial arthritis vs. reactive arthritis and rheumatoid arthritis in the adult knee. Scand J Rheumatol 1992;21: 283–8.
22. Lenski M, Scherer MA. Analysis of synovial inflammatory markers to differ infectious from gouty arthritis. Clin Biomech 2014;47:49–55.
23. Yagupsky P, Press J. Use of the isolator 1.5 microbial tube for culture of synovial fluid from patients with septic arthritis. J Clin Microbiol 1997;35:2410–2.
24. Cooper C, Cawley MI. Bacterial arthritis in an English health district: a 10-year review. Ann Rheum Dis 1986;45:458–63.
25. Sharp JT, Lidsky MD. Infectious arthritis. Arch Intern Med 1979;139:1125–30.
26. Mathews CJ, Weston VC. Bacterial septic arthritis in adults. Lancet 2010;375: 846–55.
27. Matthews PC, Dean BJ. Native hip joint septic arthritis in 20 adults: delayed presentation beyond three weeks predicts need for excision arthroplasty. J Infect 2008;57:185–90.
28. Coakley G, Mathews C, On behalf of the British Society for Rheumatology Standards, Guidelines, and Audit Working Group. BSR & BHPR, BOA, RCGP, and BSAD guidelines for the management of hot swollen joint in adults. Rheumatology 2006;45:1039–41.
29. Broy SB, Schmid FR. A comparison of medical drainage (needle aspiration) and surgical drainage (arthrotomy or arthroscopy) in the initial treatment of infected joints. Clin Rheum Dis 1986;12:501–22.
30. Maneiro JR, Souto A. Predictors of treatment failure and mortality in native septic arthritis. Clin Rheumatol 2015;34:1961–7.
31. Ravindran V, Logan I. Medical vs surgical treatment for the native joint in septic arthritis: a 6-year, single UK academic centre experience. Rheumatology 2009; 48:1320–2.
32. Harada K, McConnell I. Native joint septic arthritis: comparison of outcomes with medical and surgical management. Southern Medical Association 2019;112: 238–43.
33. Wirtz DC, Marth M. Septic arthritis of the knee in adults: treatment by arthroscopy or arthrotomy. Int Orthop 2001;25:239–41.
34. Vispo-Seara JL, Barthel T. Arthroscopic treatment of septic joints: prognostic factors. Arch Orthop Trauma Surg 2002;122:204–11.
35. Kuo CL, Chang JH. Treatment of septic knee arthritis: comparison of arthroscopic debridement alone or combined with continuous closed irrigation-suction system. J Trauma 2011;71:454–9.
36. Yanmis I, Ozkan H. The relation between the arthroscopic findings and functional outcomes in patients with septic arthritis of the knee joint, treated with arthroscopic debridement and irrigation. Acta Orthop Traumatol Turcica 2011;45:94–9.
37. Al-Nammari SS, Bobak P. Methicillin-resistant Staphylococcus aureus versus methicillin-sensitive Staphylococcus aureus adult haematogenous septic arthritis. Arch Orthop Trauma Surg 2007;127:537–42.
38. Uckay I, Tovmirzaeva L. Short parenteral antibiotic treatment for adult septic arthritis after successful drainage. Int J Infect Dis 2013;17:199–205.
39. Kodomuri P, Geutjens G. Time delay between diagnosis and arthroscopic lavage in septic arthritis. Does it matter. Int Orthop 2012;36:1727–31.

40. Lauper N, Davat M. Native septic arthritis is not an immediate surgical emergency. J Infect 2018;77:47–53.
41. Holtom PD, Borges L. Hematogenous septic ankle arthritis. Clin Orthop Relat Res 2008;466:1388–91.
42. Pioro MH, Mandell BF. Septic arthritis. Rheum Dis Clin North Am 1997;23:239–58.
43. Smith JW, Piercy EA. Infectious arthritis. Clin Infect Dis 1995;20:225–31.
44. Ferkel R. Arthroscopy of the foot and ankle. New York: Lippincott Williams & Wilkins/Raven Press; 1996.
45. Mankovecky MR, Roukis TS. Arthroscopic synovectomy, irrigation, and debridement for treatment of septic ankle arthrosis: a systematic review and case series. J Foot Ankle Surg 2014;53(5):615–9.
46. Kirchhoff C, Braunstein V. Septic arthritis as a severe complication of elective arthroscopy: clinical management strategies. Patient Saf Surg 2009;3:6.
47. Gäechter A. Der gelenkinfekt. Inform Artz 1986;6:35–43.
48. Stutz G, Kuster MS. Arthroscopic management of septic arthritis: stages of infection and results. Knee Surg Sports Traumatol Arthrosc 2000;8:270–4.
49. Boffeli TB, Thompson JC. Arthroscopic management of the septic ankle joint: case report of a stage-guided treatment. J Foot Ankle Surg 2013;52:113–7.
50. Takahashi R, Kajita Y. Factors affecting the outcome of septic arthritis of the shoulder joint with arthroscopic management. J Orthop Sci 2021;26:381–4.
51. Dave OH, Patel KA. Surgical procedures needed to eradicate infection in knee septic arthritis. Orthopedics 2016;39:50–4.

Management of Subchondral Lesions in the Foot and Ankle

Joshua Wolfe, DPM, MHA, AACFAS*, Brian Derner, DPM, AACFAS,
Ryan T. Scott, DPM, FACFAS

KEYWORDS

- Ankle arthroscopy • Subchondral lesions • Talar lesions • Bone marrow lesions
- Fragility fractures of the talus • Osteochondral lesions • Microfracture
- Calcium phosphate

KEY POINTS

- Subchondral lesions can be related to a wide variety of causes, but are primarily identified as acute trauma, repetitive microtrauma, or idiopathic means.
- Subchondral lesions associated with osteochondral lesions may be due to intravasation of synovial fluid into the subchondral bone and may lead to cystic changes.
- Treatment of these injuries should consider the cartilaginous/chondral injury as well as the subchondral injury.
- Failure to address the subchondral pathology may lead to failure of treatment or lack of resolution of symptoms for the patient.
- Treatment options for subchondral lesions includes retrograde drilling, flowable calcium phosphate, osteochondral auto/allograft transplantation, as well as en bloc allograft, among others.

INTRODUCTION

Subchondral and osteochondral lesions are challenging pathologies that the foot and ankle surgeon encounters. Osteochondritis dissecans (OCD) was first described by Konig in 1888 as a subchondral inflammatory process. His descriptions were specifically for the knee, which resulted in a loose fragment of cartilage from the femoral condyle.[1] He attributed this to 3 causes: trauma, necrosis (caused by minor trauma), or spontaneous causes. This work was furthered by Kappis in 1922, where he was the first to describe a similar pathology to the ankle.[2,3] Osteochondral lesions are treated

The CORE Institute Reconstructive Foot and Ankle Fellowship, The CORE Institute, 18444 North 25th Avenue, Suite 210, Phoenix, AZ 85023, USA
* Corresponding author. Mountainview Orthopedics, 4351 East Lohman, Suite 301, Las Cruces, NM 88011.
E-mail address: joshua.wolfe.dpm@gmail.com

Clin Podiatr Med Surg 40 (2023) 553–568
https://doi.org/10.1016/j.cpm.2023.03.005
0891-8422/23/© 2023 Elsevier Inc. All rights reserved.

podiatric.theclinics.com

through a variety of different algorithms including anterograde drilling, microfracture, abrasion chondroplasty, and osteochondral allograft/autograft transplantation, among others. The specifics of these are outside of the focus of this paper. However, management of subchondral lesions is of particular interest in this paper.

OCD must be considered through 2 different thought processes. First, as we previously mentioned, is the treatment of the cartilage injury itself. The techniques are briefly mentioned in the earlier section, which are not the focus for this article, and are addressed in an accompanying article to ours. Second is the treatment of the underlying subchondral injury to the talus. Subchondral injuries, as they pertain to osteochondral lesions of the talus (OLTs), are present due to disruption of the subchondral plate through either acute trauma, repetitive microtrauma, or idiopathic means.[4–8] Idiopathic or nontraumatic OCDs are likely due to ischemia, necrosis, and/or genetics as the primary causative factors.[7,8] As the chronicity of the injury persists, the patient becomes symptomatic through the compression of cartilage, which results in pressurization of the synovial fluid. The synovial fluid is forced into the subchondral bone through the focal injury; this occurs repetitively as cyclic loading of the ankle occurs through normal gait. This progresses to localized osteolysis and subsequent cystic changes within the subchondral bone.[8]

Conservative treatment of OLTs has been shown in minor lesions to be a reasonable treatment option. The severity and depth of the injury prognosticates the need for surgical intervention. Christensen and colleagues (1994) found that larger lesions negatively affect joint contact kinematics.[9] Klammer and colleagues (2015) found that 12% of their 43 patients with minor OLTs treated nonoperatively experienced a staged progression of their lesion.[10] Most of the patients found a decrease in lesion sizes over time (68% in width, 50% in length, and 90% in depth). Their mean lesion size at initial visit was 9.6 (W) x 8.3 (D) x 15.8 (L) mm^2, with a final follow-up size of 8.6 x 7.1 × 15.5 mm^2. It should be noted that in a systematic review by Verhagen and Van Dijk and colleagues (2003) nonsurgical treatment was successful in only 45% of cases.[11]

IMAGING

Originally, Berndt and Harty classified osteochondral defects of the talus with a 4-staged system based on plain film radiographs.[12] Since then, imaging modalities for visualization of osteochondral defects have improved. Radiographs are useful for initial evaluation of ankle pathology, but more advanced imaging has been the standard for more than 20 years. As a result, newer classification systems have been created for evidence-based treatment of OCD lesions, leading to better outcomes. As MRI quality improved, Hepple and colleagues created a classification system accounting for pathology missed on plain film radiographs.[13] They concluded that greater than 30% of osteochondral and subchondral talar lesions were missed without MRI. Their classification system (**Table 1**) labeled subchondral lesions as type V lesions. They postulated the reason these lesions occur was due to high pressure penetration of synovial fluid into the subchondral bone due to trauma of the cartilage or avascular bone present underneath an intact cartilage cap.[13]

In addition to MRI, computed axial tomography (CAT) scans have been used in evaluation of OCD lesions in the tibiotalar joint. Ferkel and colleagues created a CT staging system (**Table 2**), evaluating cystic lesions with and without intact cartilage caps.[14] For subchondral lesions, these imaging modalities are preferred to fully evaluate the extent of osteochondral injury to the tibiotalar joint. Surgeons primarily obtain MRIs for these lesions; however, MRI can overestimate the size of both subchondral cysts

Table 1
Hepple MRI classification of osteochondral lesions of the talus

Stages	Definition
1	Articular cartilage damage only
2a	Cartilage injury with underlying fracture and surrounding bony edema
2b	Stage 2a without surrounding bony edema
3	Detached but nondisplaced fragment
4	Detached and displaced fragment
5	Subchondral cyst formation

Hepple, S., Winson, I. G., & Glew, D. (1999). Osteochondral Lesions of the Talus: A Revised Classification. *Foot & Ankle International, 20*(12), 789–793. https://doi.org/10.1177/107110079902001206.

and bone marrow lesions. Recent clinical evidence showed that MRI overestimated OCD size in patients by 53.3% and undersized by 24.4%.[15] Therefore, CAT scans can be used for appropriate preoperative sizing of osteochondral lesions as well as provide further imaging to determine if there is an intact cartilage cap over a potential subchondral lesion or cyst.

The Magnetic Resonance Observation of Cartilage Repair Tissue (MOCART) was created for a standardized approach to assess cartilage lesions, specifically in the knee.[16] More recently, an updated version was created by Schreiner and colleagues to streamline some of the linguistical interpretations and increase inter- and intrarater reliability among specialists; this aided in improving consistency of scoring, which was of concern, as the reliability measures were identified as a weakness. Newer cartilage repair techniques, which will not be covered in this chapter (eg, autologous chondrocyte implantation), have necessitated a change in MOCART scores, as these techniques altered scoring.[17] The purpose of this grading system is to denote the improvement of surgical repair of the cartilage lesion. For example, in the case of a subchondral cyst greater than 5 mm in diameter, surgical correction of this cyst can improve the MOCART score by a maximum of 20 points (**Table 3**).

RETROGRADE DRILLING

When only subchondral cysts are encountered on advanced imaging, surgeons use less invasive retrograde techniques to treat these subchondral defects. The thought process of drilling in a retrograde fashion are 2-fold. First, surgeons will cause minimal damage to the intact cartilage cap and second, treatment and eradication of the

Table 2
Computed tomographic classification of osteochondral lesions of the talus by Ferkel and colleagues

Stages	Definition
I	Cystic lesion with intact roof
IIA	Cystic lesion with communication to talar dome surface
IIB	Open articular surface lesion with overlying nondisplaced fragment
III	Nondisplaced fragment with lucency
IV	Displaced fragment

Ferkel RD, Sgaglione NA, Del Pizzo W, et al. Arthroscopic treatment of osteochondral lesions of the talus: technique and results. *Orthop Trans.* 1990;14:172.

Table 3
MOCART 2.0 knee score from Schreiner et al. 2021

		Scoring
I	Volume fill of cartilage defect	
	1 Complete filling OR minor hypertrophy:100% to 150% filling of total defect volume	20
	2 Major hypertrophy $\geq$ 150% (1_2a) OR 75% to 99% filling of total defect volume (1_2b)	15
	3 50% to 74% filling of total defect volume	10
	4 25% to 49% filling of total defect volume	5
	5 < 25% filling of total defect volume (1_5a) OR complete delamination in situ (1_5b)	0
2	Integration into adjacent cartilage	
	1 Complete integration	15
	2 Split-like defect at repair tissue and native cartilage interface $\leq$ 2 mm	10
	3 Defect at repair tissue and native cartilage interface > 2 mm but <0% of repair tissue length	5
	4 Defect at repair tissue and native cartilage interface $\geq$50% of repair tissue length	0
3	Surface of the repair tissue	
	1 Surface intact	10
	2 Surface irregular < 50% of repair tissue diameter	5
	3 Surface irregular $\geq$ 50% of repair tissue diameter	0
4	Structure of the repair tissue	
	1 Homogenous	10
	2 Inhomogenous	0
5	Signal intensity of the repair tissue	
	1 Normal	15
	2 Minor abnormal-minor hyperintense (5_2a) OR minor hypointense (5_2b)	10
	3 Severely abnormal-almost fluidlike (5_3a) OR close to subchondral plate signal(5_3b)	0
6	Bony defect or bony overgrowth	
	1 No bony defect or bony overgrowth	10
	2 Bony defect: depth < thickness of adjacent cartilage (6_2a) OR overgrowth < 50% of adjacent cartilage (6_2b)	5
	3 Bony defect: depth $\geq$ thickness of adjacent cartilage (6_2a) OR overgrowth $\geq$ 50% of adjacent cartilage (6_2b)	0
7	Subchondral changes	
	1 No major subchondral changes	20
	2 Minor edema-like marrow signal-maximum diameter <50% of repair tissue diameter	15
	3 Severe edema-like marrow signal-maximum diameter $\geq$50% of repair tissue diameter	10
	4 Subchondral cyst $\geq$ 5 mm in longest diameter (7_4a) OR osteonecrosis-like signal (7_4b)	0

Abbreviation: MOCART, magnetic resonance observation of cartilage repair tissue.
Schreiner, Markus M., et al. "The MOCART (Magnetic Resonance Observation of Cartilage Repair Tissue) 2.0 Knee Score and Atlas." *CARTILAGE*, 17 Aug. 2019, p. 194760351986530, 10.1177/1947603519865308. Accessed 9 Nov. 2021.

subchondral lesion. Surgeons have also used an anterograde approach, which has been described earlier.

Taranow and colleagues were the first to describe their treatment of subchondral talar defects with retrograde autologous bone grafting. They used a cannulated drill and targeting guide to triangulate the cyst. They visualized the drilling and subsequent autografting (from the calcaneus) with both arthroscopy and intraoperative fluoroscopy to ensure no cartilage was violated. In their study of 16 ankles, with follow-up average of 2 years, they noted a mean increase in the American Orthopedic Foot and Ankle Society (AOFAS) Ankle-Hindfoot Scale score of 25 points. They also noted an 88% radiographic healing rate from this autografting without complication.[18] Retrograde drilling also showed successful outcomes in other studies, with a mean increase in AOFAS of more than 25 points.[19,20] Saxena and colleagues even illustrated an average return to activity of 7.29 months in patients receiving retrograde drilling and autografting (N = 8).[20]

Historically, anterograde drilling has been the standard for treatment of subchondral lesions. Takao and colleagues published their results on a comparative cohort study that showed an increase in the International Cartilage Repair Society (ICRS) visual repair assessment scores on second-look arthroscopy in their cohort of retrograde drilling and iliac crest autografting compared with their anterograde drilling group.[21]

In conclusion, there was a statistically significant increase in the postoperative AOFAS score of the retrograde drilling group compared with the anterograde cohort. They postulated Hepple grade V lesions should be treated with retrograde drilling compared with anterograde due to these outcomes.[21] Another comparative study was performed by Choi and Lee, which showed no statistically significant difference between their microfracture and retrograde drilling cohorts (N = 90, 40 retrograde drilling, 50 microfracture) in AOFAS, visual analog scale, and ankle activity score. However, they did note both cohorts had increases from preoperative levels in all categories.[22]

Usage of demineralized bone matrix has been studied for grafting in cases of retrograde drilling as well. Hyer and colleagues noted in their small cohort, a 34-point mean increase in AOFAS scores using this technique, with 4 of the 7 patients showing complete resolution of cysts on postoperative MRI.[23]

The International Consensus Meeting on Cartilage Repair of the Ankle created a consensus statement based on retrograde drilling. However, most of the literature that supported these statements were retrograde comparative cohort studies at best. Therefore, most of the consensus is based on weak data and more anecdotal evidence. Regardless, they had a strong consensus that retrograde drilling should be considered for isolated subchondral lesions, with or without cysts. Cancellous bone grafting is the preferred method among the consensus statement team. Bone void fillers did not have enough for or against in the treatment of these lesions. Lesions greater than 100 mm^3 should undergo bone grafting as well as drilling.[24]

There are multiple benefits to retrograde drilling compared with anterograde drilling in subchondral lesions. First, there is no damaging the overlying cartilage cap. Second, this approach allows for the delivery of autograft or allograft for direct repair of the lesion, compared with secondary repair, which is typically performed via arthroscopic picks and other anterograde techniques.[18,19,21,23] In addition, patients who have allografting of these subchondral lesions have no donor site morbidity. However, overall patient study size is lacking, regardless of modality. Therefore, higher level studies need to be performed to allow for more appropriately powered studies to improve outcomes and provide the best evidence-based treatment recommendations.

Although this treatment seems to have fewer difficulties compared with an anterograde approach, potential complications persist. Iatrogenic cartilage damage can occur if too large of a drill or overzealous drilling occur. As the talar arterial supply is very tenuous, there is the possibility of iatrogenic arterial injury to the blood supply of the talus, leading to avascular necrosis of the talus. Thermal necrosis could also occur in the incidence of sclerotic bone, aggressive drilling, or improper cooling of the drill. Without proper intraoperative radiographic triangulation, the grafting and drilling could be placed in the wrong location, which can occur up to 20%.[25]

MICROFRACTURE

Microfracture has been a main stay for smaller OLTs as a baseline measure for bone marrow stimulation. Microfracture as a treatment for OLTs has been based on the tenet of producing fibrocartilage as a replacement for the loss of hyaline cartilage seen in OLTs. Microfracture became popularized by Steadman in 2001.[26] Microfracture is performed arthroscopically with the use of a microfracture pick to disrupt the subchondral bone. The literature is clear that fibrocartilage is of lower value with regard to the biomechanical and biologic properties in comparison to hyaline cartilage.[27–29] However, replacement of hyaline cartilage with fibrocartilage has been found to be a reasonable, cost-effective alternative in lieu of alternative biological treatments. Microfracture has been established as a viable treatment option for lesions less than 150 mm^2.[27,30–36] Corr and colleagues performed a retrospective analysis of patients undergoing OLTs from 2007 to 2009 with 10 years of follow-up. They found that of their 45 respondents, only 3 required additional surgery for the OLT, and they achieved a 93.3% survivorship over that period[27]; in addition, 85.7% were able to return to sport. Furthermore, a systematic review by Dahmen and colleagues (2017) found that microfracture or bone marrow stimulation for lesions less than 15 mm were found to have a success rate of 82%.[37]

Microfracture has been hypothesized to be a contributor to subchondral lesions and cystic changes to the talus; this is largely due to the intentional disruption of the subchondral plate, which leads to the cyclic loading and pressurization of synovial fluid through the subchondral bone plate, as we have previously mentioned. Shimozono and colleagues (2017) followed-up 42 patients who underwent arthroscopic debridement with microfracture for OLTs with a mean follow-up of 51.7 months $\pm$ 22 months.[24] They followed-up these patients with a postoperative MRI as 6 to 12 months, 1 to 2 years, 2 to 4 years, and 4 to 6 years. They found that subchondral bone was not repaired at midterm follow-up and of those that underwent the fourth MRI at 4 to 6 years, 77% still had subchondral bone edema. They achieved statistical significance with regard to development of subchondral cystic changes postoperatively as well as a deteriorated subchondral bone health score; this was noted to occur between 24 and 52 months. Beck and colleagues (2016) performed a study following microfracture in sheep with follow-up CT scans and demonstrated bone cyst formation was seen in 33% of microfractured cases and 49% developed subchondral bony overgrowth. With respect to microfracture and autologous chondrocyte implantation, Beck found that subchondral bone cyst formation following cartilage repair was as high as 92% postoperatively in sheep.[38] It should be noted that this does differ from the original work of Steadman, which was studied in equine models with significantly improved results, albeit follow-up CT scans were not performed in those studies; this is in stark contrast to the results of Raikin and Corr in 2021 where they found that patients had a 93.3% (39/42) survivorship rate at 10 years as well as 85.7% (36 patients) of patients returning to sport.[27] In a separate study by Shimozono and colleagues (2018) there was found to be correlation of concomitant subchondral bone marrow edema with microfracture of OLTs to have an inferior clinical outcome in comparison to those without subchondral BME[24]; this may aid in providing some guidance in preoperative planning for surgeons considering microfracture. Controversy certainly does persist for microfracture as a treatment option for OLTs and should be carefully evaluated for cystic changes both preoperatively as well as postoperatively if microfracture is performed.

CALCIUM PHOSPHATE

Subchondral lesions to the bone, called bone marrow lesions (BMLs), are found on MRI. These lesions are seen on high-intensity T2-weighted and T1-weighted imaging.[39] The T2 images can overexaggerate the size of these BMLs, and the T1 should be used when treating these lesions intraoperatively. A theory of treatment is to stabilize osseous voids and/or gaps that may be underlying deficiencies. The thought is to rescue the intraosseous fracturing and bone resorption with a grafting substitute, creating an osteoconductive environment and structure for the body to produce new bone. BMLs are thought to be precursors to advancing cartilage destruction or joint collapse.[40] Multiple orthopedic companies have created their own proprietary version of this calcium phosphate flowable graft, the first of which was brought on to the market in 2007. Originally, studied in the knee, flowable calcium phosphate showed efficacy and positive patient outcomes with minimal complications.[39,41,42]

There has been a push to use these products in patients with BMLs (specifically the tibiotalar joint), without many studies in the foot and ankle. Beck and colleagues used a combination of core decompression with a drill and usage of a flowable calcium sulfate-calcium phosphate graft in 7 patients. They noted a statistically significant improvement in AOFAS scores from 71 to 90, primarily due to pain reduction. Beck and colleagues noted 6/7 patients having moderate daily pain originally. Following surgical decompression and grafting, 4/7 reported mild occasional daily pain, and 3/7 patients had no pain at final follow-up.[38] Other small case series have been published, showing minimal discomfort in 2 patients at more than 10 months for lesions in talus.[43]

Each BML has its own characteristics, and subsequently, the volume of bone graft substitute used for filling and treatment of lesions varies. These volumes have changed from early experience to today. Anecdotally, increased postoperative pain and avascular necrosis (AVN) of the talus have been encountered, but minimal studies have shown these results. McWilliams and colleagues, in their retrospective cohort study of 18 patients injected 1.15 cm^3 of graft into these lesions. At an average of 27.7 weeks, 3 patients improved in their symptoms, 1 patient was worse, and 4 patients were unchanged in their pain. The study also had other procedures performed with the injectable calcium phosphate, so these results may be multifactorial and do not necessarily indicate the BML repair.[44]

Newer studies have shown some adverse effects and/or complications regarding flowable calcium phosphate in several small case series. Hanselman and colleagues published a study demonstrating 7/12 patients suffered talar AVN following receiving calcium phosphate treatment of BMLs. Average time in their study for clinical suspicion of AVN was 10 months, with radiographic confirmation of 23 months on average. They did postulate that 3 of the 7 patients had prior AVN risk factors, and this could lead to a "double hit phenomena." Unfortunately, the average volume of calcium phosphate injected was not known for this study. This report had both the longest follow-up in the foot and ankle literature with regard to calcium phosphate injectables as well as the highest number of cases of AVN.[45] The evidence of AVN was furthered in another case study (Foran 2020) that performed the same treatment of BMLs but in the setting of acute lateral ankle ligament injuries. All 5 of their patients suffered talar AVN. They used calcium phosphate injectables into the talus for the bone marrow lesions, as well as repairing the lateral ankle ligament complex in 2 of the patients. On average, this cohort had clinical symptoms of AVN within 6 months. This study postulated the

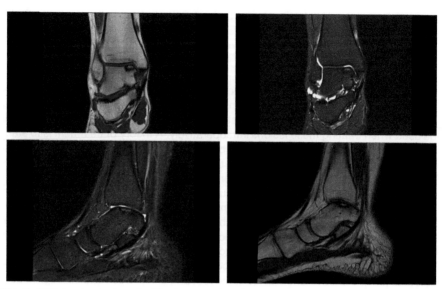

Fig. 1. MRI demonstrating significant osteochondral lesion to the medial talar dome that measured 8 × 5 × 9mm.

technique in which the surgeon used the cannula may have injured the deltoid artery (as the surgeon went from medial to lateral across the talar body). The use of calcium phosphate derivatives in an acute injury should be carefully weighed, as AVN, a potential life or limb changing complication, can occur.[46]

Surgeons must be very understanding of the power of these calcium phosphate derivatives and the possible sequelae of postoperative complications. Appropriate surgical technique, proper patient workup for AVN risk factors, as well as volume of injectable used should all be considered for optimal patient outcomes. This technology is new and lacks high-level evidence-based medicine, as there are only case studies within the literature for the ankle joint. Most of the literature for calcium phosphate injectables for BMLs is in the knee joint. These bones act differently because they are long bones, compared with the talus, which is composed of a 60% cartilaginous surface and is already predisposed to AVN in the setting of trauma. It is our opinion that care must be taken to prevent violation of the blood supply to the talus due to its tenuous perfusion and the documented risk of AVN.

When flowable calcium phosphate has been previously used, the surgeon should be aware of its depiction on advanced imaging. MRI demonstrates loss of uptake on both T1- and T2-weighted images, making the injury look worst. Flowable calcium phosphate takes time to incorporate and will be directly seen as a void in the bone. As the calcium phosphate incorporates into the talus the vascularity will eventually be demonstrated on the MRI.

BONE GRAFTING FOR SUBCHONDRAL CYSTS

Osteochondral lesions of the talus with cystic formation underlying the subchondral plate require a staged or multifaceted approach by the foot and ankle surgeon. With regard to subchondral cysts specifically, autogenous or allografting of the lesion does present as a viable option. These lesions are specifically described by Scranton

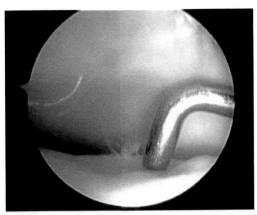

Fig. 2. Arthroscopic image of insufficiency fracture of talus with intact cartilage cap.

and McDermott as a type V osteochondral lesion.[47] Grafting of these lesions should be considered with respect to long-term staged planning for this patient population. Specifically, management of these cysts through autogenous grafting or allografting should be performed for future planning of a staged procedure rather than as an isolated procedure, as the success rate with grafting alone has been demonstrated to have poor outcomes. Kolker and colleagues (2004) performed a retrospective, consecutive review of 13 patients with advanced OCDs of the talus that underwent autologous corticocancellous bone grafting. They found that there was an overall patient satisfaction rate of 46.2% with a clinical failure rate (requiring further surgery) of 46%. However, all patients were found to have incorporation of their graft with subchondral union, which was evaluated with CT and plain radiographs.[48] Therefore, in a patient with advanced arthritis of the ankle, these patients may tolerate grafting if a staged procedure for total ankle arthroplasty is being considered.

Osteochondral autograft transplantation (OAT) is an additional option for the treatment of osteochondral lesion of the talus that addresses both chondral as well as subchondral defects of OLTs. Comparison with regard to primary and secondary lesions was studied by Park and colleagues (2018), which found similar success rates between primary and secondary lesions; this is despite a secondary OAT operation after failed initial BMS. In addition, this study specifically addressed larger lesions with a mean size of 199.2 and 190.2 mm^2 for primary and secondary lesions, respectively. It should be noted that the investigators did find that lesions greater than 225 mm^2 were found to be significantly associated with clinical failures.[49]

En bloc allograft is an additional consideration for the surgeon treating patients with unconstrained talar OLTs with subchondral cystic changes. The specifics of this will be covered in an accompanying article. However, this does remain an option in the large unconstrained lesion and requires a fresh osteochondral allograft transplantation. Albeit this treatment method does have a reported failure rate of up to 35% as well as a reoperation rate of 25% to 33%.[50–53]

CASE REPORTS
Case 1

A 23-year-old woman with 3-month history of ankle pain. She denied any history of trauma. Patient does work in a job with repetitive manual labor that requires her to walk long distances with extended-hour shifts. After failing conservative therapy,

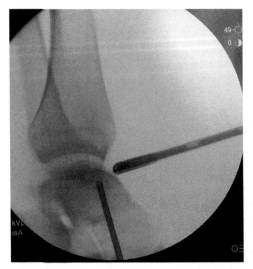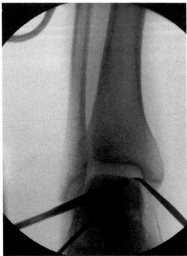

Fig. 3. Fluoroscopic triangulation of medial talar lesion with retrograde drilling and direct fluoroscopic visualization.

MRI was obtained (**Fig. 1**), which demonstrated a significant osteochondral lesion to the medial talar dome that measured 8 x 5 × 9 mm. Arthroscopy was performed to repair her OLT as well as her subchondral lesion with insufficiency fracture. Arthroscopic images can be seen in **Fig. 2**, which demonstrates her intact cartilage cap.

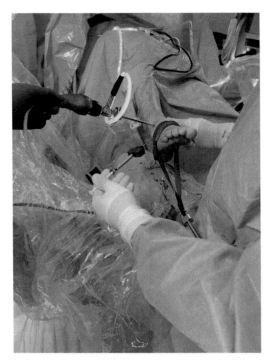

Fig. 4. Intraoperative demonstration of retrograde drilling and calcium phosphate grafting with assistant.

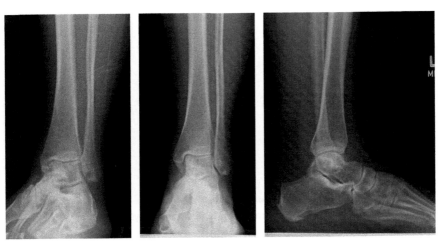

Fig. 5. Preoperative radiographs with medial talar subchondral cyst.

Retrograde drilling was then performed anterolaterally, as seen in **Fig. 3** under direct visualization arthroscopically as well as with fluoroscopy. After appropriate triangulation and placement of the cannula, flowable calcium phosphate was then injected into the insufficiency fracture, as seen in **Fig. 4**. It is our opinion that this should be done with direct visualization arthroscopically to ensure that no leakage is present within the ankle joint. After injection, the calcium phosphate is then allowed to set for the appropriate length of time as directed by the manufacturer.

Case 2

The patient is a 46-year-old woman who initially presented as a second opinion regarding persistent ankle pain despite several surgeries to her ankle. She initially injured her ankle in a snowboarding accident. She presented after a history of multiple arthroscopies including calcium phosphate treatment of a subchondral lesion and an OCD repair with microfracture. Preoperative radiographs can be seen in **Fig. 5**. MRI and CT were performed and can be seen in **Figs. 6** and **7**, respectively. Her MRI and CT demonstrated a large osteochondral lesion of the talar dome as well as persistent calcium phosphate material retained within the shoulder of the talus. She was also noted to have posttraumatic tibiotalar osteoarthrosis with cartilage loss and cystic

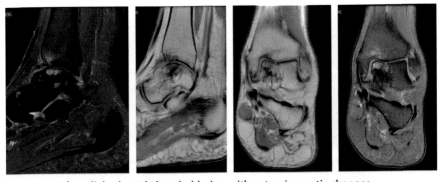

Fig. 6. MRI of medial talar subchondral lesion with extensive cystic changes.

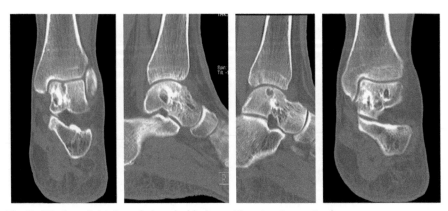

Fig. 7. CT of medial talar subchondral lesion with extensive cystic changes.

changes within the medial shoulder of the talus. Surgical intervention was performed after appropriate failure of conservative therapy and in conjunction with the patient's goals with anticipated staging for future procedures. The patient underwent ankle arthroscopy with proximal tibial autograft harvesting and retrograde drilling with

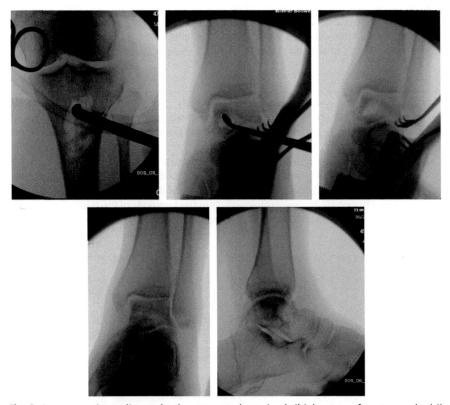

Fig. 8. Intraoperative radiographs demonstrated proximal tibial autograft, retrograde drilling with curettage of the talus from an anterolateral approach, and grafting with proximal tibial autograft and rhBMP-2.

curettage from the anterolateral aspect of the talus with combined autografting and biological augmentation using rhBMP-2 in an absorbable collagen sponge carrier seen in **Fig. 8**.

SUMMARY

Management of subchondral lesions has a variety of treatment options to be considered. Proper application of techniques with appropriate patient selection is paramount to attain acceptable surgical outcomes. The literature has demonstrated that there is a correlation between microfracture of the subchondral bone plate and the development of subchondral lesions. Intuitively, treatment of smaller lesions has been demonstrated to have improved outcomes compared with larger end-stage lesions; this is seen through the poorer outcomes of larger allograft procedures.

CLINICS CARE POINTS

- When evaluating osteochondral lesions, care should be taken to evaluate for subchondral lesions and cystic changes.
- When performing advanced imaging for evaluation of osteochondral lesions, be aware of the ability of MRI to overestimate lesion size. One should consider CT evaluation for osteochondral lesions, as well as for all subchondral lesions.
- When performing arthroscopic repair of OLTs, one should be aware of the risk of subchondral cystic changes with microfracture. One should consider arthroscopic abrasion chondroplasty with grafting, if indicated.
- Management of subchondral lesions with calcium phosphate must be performed carefully to avoid development of AVN. One should be aware of the postoperative changes on MRI with calcium phosphate products, as it presents similarly on MRI as AVN.

ACKNOWLEDGMENTS

Thank you to Dr Jeffrey Holmes, DPM for his contribution of his case report for this paper.

DISCLOSURE

Drs J. Wolfe, B. Derner, and R.T. Scott have no conflicts to disclose pertaining to this paper.

REFERENCES

1. König F. [About free body in the joints][in German]. Zeiteschr Chir 1888;27: 90–109.
2. Kappis M. Weitere Beiträge zur traumatisch-mechanischen Entstehung der "spontanen" Knorpelablösungen (sogen. Osteochondritis dissecans). Deutsche Zeitschrift für Chirurgie 1922;171(1):13–29.
3. Zanon G, G DIV, Marullo M. Osteochondritis dissecans of the talus. Joints 2014; 2(3):115–23.
4. Bruns J. [Osteochondrosis dissecans]. Orthopade 1997;26(6):573–84. Osteochondrosis dissecans.
5. Ray RB, Coughlin EJ Jr. Osteochondritis dissecans of the talus. J Bone Joint Surg Am 1947;29(3):697–706.

6. Reilingh M, Van Bergen C, Van Dijk C. Diagnosis and treatment of osteochondral defects of the ankle. SA Orthopaedic Journal 2009;8(2):44–50.
7. Schachter AK, Chen AL, Reddy PD, et al. Osteochondral lesions of the talus. JAAOS-Journal of the American Academy of Orthopaedic Surgeons 2005; 13(3):152–8.
8. van Dijk CN, Reilingh ML, Zengerink M, et al. Osteochondral defects in the ankle: why painful? Knee Surg Sports Traumatol Arthrosc 2010;18(5):570–80.
9. Christensen JC, Driscoll HL, Tencer AF. 1994 William J. Stickel Gold Award. Contact characteristics of the ankle joint. Part 2. The effects of talar dome cartilage defects. J Am Podiatr Med Assoc 1994;84(11):537–47.
10. Klammer G, Maquieira GJ, Spahn S, et al. Natural history of nonoperatively treated osteochondral lesions of the talus. Foot Ankle Int 2015;36(1):24–31.
11. Verhagen RA, Struijs PA, Bossuyt PM, et al. Systematic review of treatment strategies for osteochondral defects of the talar dome. Foot Ankle Clin 2003;8(2): 233–42, viii-ix.
12. Berndt AL, Harty M. Transchondral fractures (osteochondritis dissecans) of the talus. J Bone Joint Surg Am 1959;41-a:988–1020.
13. Hepple S, Winson IG, Glew D. Osteochondral lesions of the talus: a revised classification. Foot Ankle Int 1999;20(12):789–93.
14. Ferkel R, Sgaglione N, DelPizzo W. Arthroscopic treatment of osteochondral lesions of the talus: long-term results. Orthop Trans 1990;14:172–3.
15. Yasui Y, Hannon CP, Fraser EJ, et al. Lesion size measured on MRI does not accurately reflect arthroscopic measurement in talar osteochondral lesions. Orthop J Sports Med 2019;7(2). 2325967118825261.
16. Marlovits S, Singer P, Zeller P, et al. Magnetic resonance observation of cartilage repair tissue (MOCART) for the evaluation of autologous chondrocyte transplantation: determination of interobserver variability and correlation to clinical outcome after 2 years. Eur J Radiol 2006;57(1):16–23.
17. Schreiner MM, Raudner M, Marlovits S, et al. The MOCART (magnetic resonance observation of cartilage repair tissue) 2.0 knee score and Atlas. Cartilage 2021; 13(1_suppl):571s–87s.
18. Taranow WS, Bisignani GA, Towers JD, et al. Retrograde drilling of osteochondral lesions of the medial talar dome. Foot Ankle Int 1999;20(8):474–80.
19. Anders S, Lechler P, Rackl W, et al. Fluoroscopy-guided retrograde core drilling and cancellous bone grafting in osteochondral defects of the talus. Int Orthop 2012;36(8):1635–40.
20. Saxena A, Maffulli N, Jin A, et al. Outcomes of talar osteochondral and transchondral lesions using an algorithmic approach based on size, location, and subchondral plate integrity: a 10-year study on 204 lesions. J Foot Ankle Surg 2022;61(3): 442–7.
21. Takao M, Innami K, Komatsu F, et al. Retrograde cancellous bone plug transplantation for the treatment of advanced osteochondral lesions with large subchondral lesions of the ankle. Am J Sports Med. Aug 2010;38(8):1653–60.
22. Choi JI, Lee KB. Comparison of clinical outcomes between arthroscopic subchondral drilling and microfracture for osteochondral lesions of the talus. Knee Surg Sports Traumatol Arthrosc 2016;24(7):2140–7.
23. Hyer CF, Berlet GC, Philbin TM, et al. Retrograde drilling of osteochondral lesions of the talus. Foot Ankle Spec 2008;1(4):207–9.
24. Shimozono Y, Brown AJ, Batista JP, et al. Subchondral pathology: proceedings of the international consensus meeting on cartilage repair of the ankle. Foot Ankle Int 2018;39(1_suppl):48s–53s.

25. Citak M, Kendoff D, Kfuri M Jr, et al. Accuracy analysis of Iso-C3D versus fluoroscopy-based navigated retrograde drilling of osteochondral lesions: a pilot study. J Bone Joint Surg Br 2007;89(3):323–6.

26. Steadman JR, Rodkey WG, Rodrigo JJ. Microfracture: surgical technique and rehabilitation to treat chondral defects. Clin Orthop Relat Res 2001;(391 Suppl):S362–9. https://doi.org/10.1097/00003086-200110001-00033.

27. Corr D, Raikin J, O'Neil J, et al. Long-term outcomes of microfracture for treatment of osteochondral lesions of the talus. Foot Ankle Int 2021;42(7):833–40.

28. Mankin HJ. The response of articular cartilage to mechanical injury. J Bone Joint Surg Am 1982;64(3):460–6.

29. Gobbi A, Francisco RA, Lubowitz JH, et al. Osteochondral lesions of the talus: randomized controlled trial comparing chondroplasty, microfracture, and osteochondral autograft transplantation. Arthroscopy 2006;22(10):1085–92.

30. Amendola A, Panarella L. Osteochondral lesions: medial versus lateral, persistent pain, cartilage restoration options and indications. Foot Ankle Clin 2009;14(2): 215–27.

31. Choi WJ, Park KK, Kim BS, et al. Osteochondral lesion of the talus: is there a critical defect size for poor outcome? Am J Sports Med 2009;37(10):1974–80.

32. Giannini S, Vannini F. Operative treatment of osteochondral lesions of the talar dome: current concepts review. Foot Ankle Int. Mar 2004;25(3):168–75.

33. Chuckpaiwong B, Berkson EM, Theodore GH. Microfracture for osteochondral lesions of the ankle: outcome analysis and outcome predictors of 105 cases. Arthroscopy 2008;24(1):106–12.

34. Lahm A, Erggelet C, Steinwachs M, et al. Arthroscopic management of osteochondral lesions of the talus: results of drilling and usefulness of magnetic resonance imaging before and after treatment. Arthroscopy 2000;16(3):299–304.

35. van Bergen CJ, de Leeuw PA, van Dijk CN. Treatment of osteochondral defects of the talus. Rev Chir Orthop Reparatrice Appar Mot 2008;94(8 Suppl):398–408.

36. van Dijk CN, van Bergen CJ. Advancements in ankle arthroscopy. J Am Acad Orthop Surg 2008;16(11):635–46.

37. Dahmen J, Lambers KTA, Reilingh ML, et al. No superior treatment for primary osteochondral defects of the talus. Knee Surg Sports Traumatol Arthrosc 2018; 26(7):2142–57.

38. Beck A, Murphy DJ, Carey-Smith R, et al. Treatment of articular cartilage defects with microfracture and autologous matrix-induced chondrogenesis leads to extensive subchondral bone cyst formation in a sheep model. Am J Sports Med 2016;44(10):2629–43.

39. Bonadio MB, Giglio PN, Helito CP, et al. Subchondroplasty for treating bone marrow lesions in the knee - initial experience. Rev Bras Ortop 2017;52(3): 325–30.

40. Wluka AE, Wang Y, Davies-Tuck M, et al. Bone marrow lesions predict progression of cartilage defects and loss of cartilage volume in healthy middle-aged adults without knee pain over 2 yrs. Rheumatology 2008;47(9):1392–6.

41. Chua K, Kang JYB, Ng FDJ, et al. Subchondroplasty for bone marrow lesions in the arthritic knee results in pain relief and improvement in function. J Knee Surg 2021;34(6):665–71.

42. Ververidis AN, Paraskevopoulos K, Tilkeridis K, et al. Surgical modalities for the management of bone marrow edema of the knee joint. J Orthop 2020;17:30–7.

43. Miller JR, Dunn KW. Subchondroplasty of the ankle: a novel technique. Foot Ankle Online J 2015;8(1):1–7.

44. McWilliams GD, Yao L, Simonet LB, et al. Subchondroplasty of the ankle and hindfoot for treatment of osteochondral lesions and stress fractures: initial imaging experience. Foot Ankle Spec 2020;13(4):306–14.

45. Hanselman AE, Cody EA, Easley ME, et al. Avascular necrosis of the talus after subchondroplasty. Foot Ankle Int 2021;42(9):1138–43.

46. Foran IM, Bohl DD, Vora AM, et al. Talar osteonecrosis after subchondroplasty for acute lateral ligament injuries: case series. Foot Ankle Orthop 2020;1. 2473011420907072.

47. Scranton PE Jr, McDermott JE. Treatment of type V osteochondral lesions of the talus with ipsilateral knee osteochondral autografts. Foot Ankle Int 2001;22(5): 380–4.

48. Kolker D, Murray M, Wilson M. Osteochondral defects of the talus treated with autologous bone grafting. Journal of Bone and Joint Surgery British 2004;86(4): 521–6.

49. Park KH, Hwang Y, Han SH, et al. Primary versus secondary osteochondral autograft transplantation for the treatment of large osteochondral lesions of the talus. Am J Sports Med 2018;46(6):1389–96.

50. Juels CA, So E, Seidenstricker C, et al. Complications of en bloc osteochondral talar allografts and treatment of failures: literature review and case report. J Foot Ankle Surg 2020;59(1):149–55.

51. Gross AE, Agnidis Z, Hutchison CR. Osteochondral defects of the talus treated with fresh osteochondral allograft transplantation. Foot Ankle Int 2001;22(5): 385–91.

52. VanTienderen RJ, Dunn JC, Kusnezov N, et al. Osteochondral allograft transfer for treatment of osteochondral lesions of the talus: a systematic review. Arthrosc J Arthrosc Relat Surg 2017;33(1):217–22.

53. Pomajzl RJ, Baker EA, Baker KC, et al. Case series with histopathologic and radiographic analyses following failure of fresh osteochondral allografts of the talus. Foot Ankle Int 2016;37(9):958–67.

Moving?

Make sure your subscription moves with you!

To notify us of your new address, find your **Clinics Account Number** (located on your mailing label above your name), and contact customer service at:

Email: journalscustomerservice-usa@elsevier.com

800-654-2452 (subscribers in the U.S. & Canada)
314-447-8871 (subscribers outside of the U.S. & Canada)

Fax number: 314-447-8029

Elsevier Health Sciences Division
Subscription Customer Service
3251 Riverport Lane
Maryland Heights, MO 63043

*To ensure uninterrupted delivery of your subscription, please notify us at least 4 weeks in advance of move.